KW-220-031

PREFACE TO THE SECOND EDITION

The opportunity has been taken in this new edition to improve some of the Figures and to include a few new ones. At the same time some omissions in the text have been rectified and an attempt has been made to clarify some of the explanations and to emphasize the general biological significance of immune phenomena.

I am most grateful to my colleague Dr Andrew Fraser for providing a critical appraisal of the text of the first edition and to many of my colleagues for useful suggestions arising from the use of the book for teaching purposes.

1971   D. M. WEIR

IMMUNOLOGY
FOR UNDERGRADUATES

The Author

D. M. WEIR, M.D. (Edin.)

Immunology Laboratory, Department of Bacteriology
University of Edinburgh Medical School

Immunology
for Undergraduates

D. M. WEIR

SECOND EDITION

CHURCHILL LIVINGSTONE
EDINBURGH AND LONDON
1971

© LONGMAN GROUP LIMITED, 1971

*All rights reserved. No part of this pub-
lication may be reproduced, stored in a
retrieval system, or transmitted in any form
or by any means, electronic, mechanical,
photocopying, recording or otherwise, without the prior permission of the publishers
E. & S. Livingstone, Teviot Place,
Edinburgh*

ISBN 0 443 00826 4

FIRST EDITION 1970
SECOND EDITION 1971

Filmset by Typesetting Services Ltd. Glasgow
and printed offset by T. & A. Constable,
Hopetoun Street, Edinburgh

PREFACE TO THE FIRST EDITION

This short survey of Immunology is derived in the main from lecture material prepared for medical students in the paraclinical stage of their course and for science undergraduates in third year microbiology. The aim of the book is to provide a short text suitable for undergraduates not necessarily intending to specialize in Immunology but who wish to be familiar with the general principles of immunological phenomena and their wide ranging relevance in biology and medicine. For those who may perhaps be stimulated to delve more deeply into the subject there are a number of excellent modern textbooks, including *Immunology for Students of Medicine, Immunology in Clinical Medicine, Structural Concepts in Immunology and Immunochemistry* and *Clinical Aspects of Immunology* for the more advanced students of medicine. These are included in the suggestions for further reading at the end of individual chapters. The text itself in the interests of clarity and simplicity contains no references. The names of individuals associated with particular areas of work are omitted except where they are associated with a phenomenon by common usage.

The Figures are, in the main, highly simplified views of complex situations and the hope is that accuracy has not been sacrificed for clarity.

I am extremely grateful to my colleague Mr W. H. McBride for reading the manuscript and for providing valuable constructive criticism of the text. The Figures were kindly prepared by the late Mr T. C. Dodds of the Medical Photography Department and Mr John Pizer of his staff gave much help in preparing the drawings. My thanks are due to the publishers for their co-operation in producing the text and particularly to my colleague Dr R. R. Gillies for checking the manuscript and for his advice and encouragement in the writing of the book.

1970   D. M. WEIR

CONTENTS

Chapter 1

IMMUNITY

The Scope of Immunology

The tissues and cells capable of exhibiting what is now recognized as an adaptive immune response have an evolutionary history of some 400 million years and the forms taken by the response during this period have maintained a remarkable constancy both at the molecular and the functional level. The meaning of the term 'immunity' as it is used today derives from its earlier usage referring to exemption from military service or paying taxes. It has long been recognized that those who recovered from epidemic diseases such as smallpox and plague were exempt from further attacks and such immune individuals were often used in an epidemic to nurse those suffering from active disease. In England the procedure of cow-pox vaccination developed by Edward Jenner in 1798 for protection against smallpox and that used by Francis Home in Edinburgh for measles protection were essentially empirical measures performed without understanding of the underlying principles. The foundations for an understanding of immunity were laid by the invention of the microscope, the recognition of microorganisms and the advent of Pasteur's germ theory of disease. Pasteur's chance observation that aged cultures of chicken cholera bacillus would not cause the expected disease in chickens led to the development of methods for reducing the virulence of pathogenic microorganisms called attenuation. The protection given to animals by pre-inoculation of such attenuated organisms led to the widespread use of the method for immunization purposes. Immunology as a science began with the demonstration by von Behring and Kitasato at the Koch Institute in Berlin in 1890 of an anti-bacterial substance or factor in the blood of animals immunized against tetanus and diphtheria organisms. The neutralizing ability of such blood serum for the bacterial toxins was the first demonstration of the effect of what is now recognized as antibody globulin.

The part played by phagocytic cells in clearing away and destroying bacteria was recognized by Metchnikoff, a Russian biologist working in France. Later the helpful effect of antibody (called opsonins by Almroth Wright) in encouraging phagocytosis became apparent thus reconciling two opposing schools of thought on immune mechanisms – one believing the process to be brought about completely by blood factors and the other upholding an entirely cellular viewpoint.

The specificity of antibody for the agent (i.e. the antigen) which induced its formation led to the use of antibody as an analytic tool. Thus the antigenic characters of bacterial and non-bacterial substances could be worked out and systems of classification of microorganisms were developed on this basis. Landsteiner used antibody-antigen interaction to define the ABO blood group system on the basis of antigenic differences in red cell membranes, and was also responsible for performing the ground work on the chemical basis of antigenic specificity.

In more recent years with increasing knowledge of the molecular processes underlying the functioning of cells it became possible to formulate theories on the mechanisms whereby the tissues and cells responsible for producing antibody performed this function. The need for such theories became apparent with the recognition of human diseases where the immune mechanisms had become deranged and were treating the individual's own tissues as if they were foreign antigens. Thus the question of how the immune system distinguished between what was foreign and what was part of self became important and resulted in the formulation of new theories to explain these phenomena, notable among which was the clonal selection theory of Burnet. These attempted to define the scope and limitation of Ehrlich's 'contrivances by means of which the immunity reaction .... is prevented from acting against the organism's own elements and so giving rise to autotoxin'. The advances made in this area gave a new dimension to the science of immunology which until then was devoted almost exclusively to the prevention of infectious disease by vaccination and immunization. This new field of study – immunobiology – has drawn the attention of biologists to the apparent central importance of immune mechanisms in the evolution of multicellular animals. Knowledge of the genetic control of protein synthesis is likely to make considerable advances as a result of the study of the synthesis of immunoglobulins.

Modern biochemical techniques have helped to add precision and sensitivity to immunological methods. These include the use of radioisotopes to measure accurately the primary binding of antibody with antigen and to demonstrate the metabolic activity of cells engaged in antibody production. Protein fractionation techniques and peptide analysis of the antibody molecule have thrown light on the chemical basis of specificity of the molecule and the relationship of structure to function as well as confirming a genetic basis for antibody formation and providing factual limitations on earlier theories of antibody formation. The understanding of immunological processes underlying the reaction of the body to tumours, to transplanted tissues and organs and to infectious agents has gained much ground as the result of these advances in immunochemical techniques. Clinical developments have included the recognition of autoimmune and immunological deficiency diseases and the feasibility of organ transplantation. Phylogenetic studies have stimulated investigations into the development and control of the lymphoid tissues leading for example to a new understanding of the role of that previously enigmatic organ, the thymus.

Thus it can be seen that immunity in its original meaning, referring to resistance to invasion by a parasite by means of a specific immune response is only one activity of a cellular system in animals the total activity of which is concerned with mechanisms for preserving the integrity of the individual with far-reaching implications in embryology, genetics, cell biology, tumour biology and many non-infective disease processes.

The subject of immunology can be considered under three general headings: immunity, dealing with the adaptive response to infective agents; immunochemistry, concerned with the chemical nature of antigens and antibodies; and immunobiology, which encompasses a variety of topics of biological importance and deals with the activity of the cells of the immune system and their relationship to each other and their environment.

Chapter 2

INNATE IMMUNITY:
NON-SPECIFIC DEFENCE MECHANISMS

The healthy individual is able to protect himself from potentially harmful microorganisms in the environment by a number of very effective mechanisms present from birth which do not depend upon having previous experience of any particular microorganism. The innate immune mechanisms are non-specific in the sense that they are effective against a wide range of potentially infective agents. The main determinants of innate immunity seem genetically controlled, varying widely with species and strain and to a lesser extent between individuals. Age, sex and hormone balance play lesser roles. In comparison, acquired immune mechanisms, discussed below, depend upon the development of an immune response to individual microorganisms that is specific only for the inducing organism.

Determinants of Innate Immunity

Species and strain

Marked differences exist in the susceptibility of different species to infective agents. The rat is strikingly insusceptible to diphtheria whilst the guinea-pig and man are highly susceptible. The rabbit is particularly susceptible to myxomatosis and man to syphilis, leprosy and meningococcal meningitis. Susceptibility to an infection does not always imply a lack of resistance because although man is highly susceptible to the common cold he overcomes the infection within a few days. Dogs in contrast are not susceptible to the virus agents responsible for the common cold in man. In some diseases, although a species may be difficult to infect (i.e. insusceptible), once established the disease can progress rapidly (i.e. lack of resistance). For example rabies

4

although common to both man and dogs is not readily established as the virus does not easily penetrate healthy skin. Once infected, however, the resistance mechanisms in both species are not able to overcome the disease. Marked variations in resistance to infection between different strains of mice have been noted.

In man the habits and environment of a community affect its ability to resist particular infections by acquired immune mechanisms developing early in life. This environmentally determined type of resistance is easily confused with the genetically

Table 1 Determinants of innate immunity

Specific host determinants	*Physical determinants*	*Active anti-microbial determinants*
Species and strain	Skin and mucous membrane barriers, moist surfaces	Anti-bacterial and anti-fungal secretions of skin – sweat and sebaceous secretions
Individual genetic factors	Anatomical traps, e.g. nasal cavity	
Age	Mechanical cleansing, e.g. cilia	Anti-bacterial and anti-viral secretions of mucous membranes
Hormonal balance		Anti-microbial substances of tissue fluids, e.g. lysozyme, basic polypeptides Phagocytosis and digestion

controlled innate immunity and makes it difficult to establish differences in innate immunity in different communities. It is however fairly clear that the American Indian and the Negro are more susceptible to tuberculosis than are Caucasians. It seems reasonable to assume that certain interspecies and interstrain differences have arisen by a process of natural selection.

Individual differences and influence of age

The role of heredity in determining resistance to infection is well illustrated by studies on tuberculosis infection in twins. If

5

one homozygous twin develops tuberculosis, the other twin has a three to one chance of developing the disease compared to a one in three chance if the twins are heterozygous. Sometimes genetically controlled abnormalities are an advantage to the individual in resisting infection as for example in a hereditary abnormality of the red blood cells (sickling) which are not able to be parasitized by *Plasmodium falciparum* thus conferring insusceptibility to malaria. Infectious diseases are more severe at the extremes of life, and in the young animal this appears to be associated with immaturity of the immunological mechanisms affecting the ability of the lymphoid system to deal with and react to foreign antigens. In the elderly on the other hand physical abnormalities (e.g. prostatic enlargement leading to stasis of urine) are a common cause of increased susceptibility to infection.

Sex and hormonal influences

There is decreased resistance to infection in diseases such as diabetes mellitus, hypothyroidism and adrenal dysfunction. The reasons for this have yet to be elucidated in detail but it is known that the glucocorticoids are anti-inflammatory agents, decreasing the ability of phagocytes to digest ingested material (probably by stabilizing the lysozome membranes). They also have the beneficial effect of interfering in some way with the toxic effects of bacterial products such as bacterial endotoxin.

There are not marked differences in susceptibility to infection between sexes but both infectious hepatitis and whooping cough have a higher morbidity and mortality in females than in males, although the overall morbidity from infectious diseases is greater in the male than in the female.

Mechanisms of Innate Immunity

Mechanical barriers and surface secretions

The intact skin and mucous membranes of the body afford effective protection against non-pathogenic organisms and a high degree of protection against pathogens (Fig. 1). The skin is the more resistant barrier because of its outer horny layer. The damp surface of the mucous membranes of the respiratory tract acts as

Fig. 1 Innate immune mechanisms

SKIN

RESPIRATORY MUCOUS MEMBRANE

Cilia
Epithelium
Muscle layer
Gland

Secretions --- Moist surface bactericidal and viricidal secretions

Antifungal and antibacterial sebaceous secretions and sweat

Mechanical barrier

Phagocytic cells

Antibacterial substances in tissue fluids

Initiates acquired immunity

Sweat gland
Sebaceous gland

Stratum corneum

Hair follicle

a trapping mechanism and together with the action of the hair-like processes or cilia, sweep away foreign particulate material so that it passes into the saliva and then is swallowed. On reaching the stomach the acid gastric juices destroy any microorganisms present. Nasal secretions and saliva contain mucopolysaccharides capable of inactivating some viruses and the tears contain lysozyme active against Gram-positive bacteria. The sebaceous secretions and sweat of the skin contain bactericidal and fungicidal fatty acids and these constitute a very effective protective mechanism against potentially pathogenic microorganisms. Certain areas of the body such as the soles of the feet are deficient in sebaceous glands and this explains in part why such areas are susceptible to fungal infection. The protective ability of these secretions varies at different stages of life and it is known that fungal 'ringworm' infection of children disappears at puberty.

Bactericidal substances of the tissues and body fluids

Lysozyme

This is a low molecular weight basic protein found in relatively high concentration in polymorphonuclear leucocytes as well in most tissue fluids except CSF, sweat and urine. It functions as a mucolytic enzyme, splitting sugars off the glycopeptides of the cell wall of many Gram-positive bacteria and resulting in their lysis. Lysozyme may also play a role in the intracellular destruction of some Gram-negative bacteria. This antibacterial agent was described by Fleming in 1922 who was able to measure its effect on a particular Gram-positive organism *Micrococcus lysodeikticus*. Human tears contain a large quantity of lysozyme and egg white is a rich commercial source.

Basic polypeptides

A variety of basic proteins, derived from the tissue and blood cells damaged in the course of infection and inflammation, have been found in the tissues of animals. This group includes spermine and spermidine, which kill tubercle bacilli and some staphylococci, and the arginine and lysine containing basic proteins protamine and histone. The ability of these basic polypeptides to destroy bacteria probably depends on their ability to react non-specifically with the nearest acidic substance.

Phagocytosis and the inflammatory response

Microorganisms or inert particles such as colloidal carbon entering the tissue fluids or blood stream are very rapidly engulfed by various circulating and tissue-fixed phagocytic cells. These cells are of two types, the polymorphonuclear leucocytes of the blood – or microphages as they are sometimes called – and the mononuclear phagocytic cells distributed throughout the body both circulating in the blood and fixed in the tissues. The latter cells make up the cells of the reticuloendothelial system or RES and are given the generic name macrophages. Macrophages in the blood are known as monocytes, those in the connective tissues as histiocytes, those in the spleen, lymph nodes and thymus as the sinus-lining macrophages (sometimes called reticulum cells). It is now established that the macrophages of connective tissues are derived from peripheral blood monocytes as are the Kupffer cells of the liver, the alveolar macrophages of the lungs, and the free macrophages of the spleen, lymph nodes and bone marrow. In the spleen and lymph nodes, both free and fixed macrophages occur in close association with the reticular cells which act as a framework for the macrophages. The reticular cells themselves although able to ingest particulate material are not regarded as mononuclear phagocytes nor are the dendritic cells (p. 50) of the follicles of the spleen and lymph nodes. The term *mononuclear phagocyte system* to describe actively phagocytic cells is now gaining favour as a more satisfactory description of the function, origin and morphology of phagocytes than the older RES classification which included actively and poorly phagocytic cells.

The three essential features of these phagocytic cells are (1) that they are actively phagocytic, (2) that they contain digestive enzymes to degrade ingested material and (3) that the macrophages are an important link between the innate and the acquired immune mechanisms, partly by passing on antigens or their products to the lymphoid cells and partly by retaining antigens to ensure that lymphoid cells are not overwhelmed by excess antigen (p. 50).

The process of phagocytosis is undoubtedly one of the earliest accomplishments of living cells. At the beginning of the century

Metchnikoff in Russia first appreciated the continuity of this function through evolution and the important role of this activity in resistance to infectious agents.

The role of the phagocyte in innate immunity is to engulf particulate (phagocytosis) or soluble material (pinocytosis) and either to digest it or if indigestible to store it away so that it no longer serves as a local irritant, e.g. carbon particles from a polluted atmosphere.

The macrophages of the reticulo-endothelial system serve a very important role in clearing the blood stream of foreign particulate material such as bacteria. The efficiency of this process can be dramatically illustrated by injecting colloidal carbon into the circulation of a mouse. Samples of blood taken at short intervals thereafter show a very rapid removal of most of the particles within a few minutes after injection and the blood is completely cleared by 15–20 minutes. Dissection of the animal will show massive localization of the carbon particles, particularly in Kupffer cells of the liver, of the spleen sinus-lining macrophages and in the macrophages of the lungs. This system of phagocytic cells has an enormous capacity to take up material from the blood and the finding of free microorganisms in the blood stream usually means that there is a continued release of organisms from an abscess or from the bacterial 'vegetation' found in bacterial endocarditis.

There are many examples of the ability of the phagocytic cells of animals to ingest and dispose of different kinds of microorganisms. The destruction of phagocytic cells by chemical agents in the rabbit results in the animal losing resistance to a normally avirulent pneumococcus. The enhanced ability of macrophages from animals infected with tubercle bacilli or listeria to resist these and other infective agents is discussed on page 94. Some microorganisms such as brucellae and streptococci can resist intracellular digestion (p. 93).

Phagocytosis can occur in the absence of serum antibodies especially on surfaces such as lung alveoli. On the other hand antibodies can markedly enhance the activities of phagocytic cells and even improve intracellular digestion. Such antibodies are known as opsonins (p. 47). Injury to tissue excites an inflammatory response consisting of dilation of local capillaries, slowing of the blood flow and exudation of oedema fluid, and phagocytic cells which initially stick to capillary walls then pass through the walls of these more permeable vessels. Once outside the capillaries the phagocytic cells, which are initially mainly the polymorphonuclear leucocytes of the blood, migrate to the source of the irritation. This leucocyte attraction phenomenon is known as chemotaxis and can readily be induced by micro-organisms entering the tissues, by the breakdown products of damaged tissue cells and by various irritant substances (possibly acting in this way because they bring about damage to cells). The precise mechanisms of chemotaxis are not understood but it is known that complexes of antigen and antibody generate the production of a diffusible factor which also acts in this way; this phenomenon requires the participation of complement components (p. 12).

After the initial polymorph infiltration in an inflammatory response, the mononuclear cells (blood macrophages) can be seen to enter the area but very little is known at present about the nature of the mechanisms which lead to the accumulation of these cells. The process seems to be quite distinct from that responsible for polymorph migration.

Once ingested, susceptible bacteria disintegrate within an hour or two partly because of the secretion of acids and digestive enzymes secreted into the vacuole surrounding them. The cytoplasmic granules (lysosomes) of polymorphs contain many enzymes including acid and alkaline phosphatase, β glucuronidase and ribonuclease. The antibacterial agents lysozyme (p. 8) and phagocytin are also present. These cytoplasmic granules fuse with the vacuole containing the microorganism.

Phagocytin

Extracts of the cytoplasm of polymorphonuclear leucocytes from several species have been found to contain an acid soluble protein bactericidal to Gram-negative bacteria and also to a few Gram-positive organisms. Phagocytin is present together with other antibacterial substances in the granules of polymorphs.

Temperature

The temperature dependence of many microorganisms is well known and tubercle bacilli, pathogenic for mammalian species, will not infect cold-blooded animals. Hens which are naturally

11

immune to anthrax can be infected if their temperature is lowered. Gonococci are readily killed at temperatures over 40°C and fever therapy was a common treatment of gonococcal infection before the introduction of antibiotics.

It is therefore apparent that temperature is an important factor in determining the innate immunity of an animal to some infective agents and it seems likely that the pyrexia which follows so many different types of infection can function as a protective response against the infecting microorganisms.

The Complement System

The existence of a heat labile serum component with the ability to lyse red blood cells and destroy Gram-negative bacteria has been known for the last 50 years or so. The chemical complexity of the phenomenon was not initially appreciated by early workers who ascribed the activity to a single component – *complement*. It is now known that complement is in fact an extremely complex group of serum proteins present in low concentration in normal serum. Collectively the complement system is the effector mechanism responsible for the biological activity of complement-fixing antibodies (p. 46).

Complement components have the characteristic of interacting with certain antibody molecules once these have combined with antigen. These components are best known for their ability to combine with anti-erythrocyte antibody attached to the red cell membrane, the effect of complement being to bring about lysis of the red cell by what appears to be enzymic digestion of small areas of the cell membrane. Much of what is known today about the complement system comes from studies of immune haemolysis.

The erythrocyte (E) – usually sheep red cells – is coated with rabbit anti-sheep red cell antibody (A). These 'sensitized' erythrocytes (EA) react with the first component of complement (C′ 1). C′ 1 is a trimolar complex high molecular weight (700,000) globulin existing in serum as an enzyme precursor. The three components of the complex are held together by calcium ions and are known as C′ 1q, C′ 1r and C′ 1s. They can be separated by chromatography and gel filtration methods. The C′ 1q component combines with a receptor on the antibody molecule. The inability of some immunoglobulins (e.g. IgA,

p. 45) to activate complement is due to the absence of the appropriate receptor. The precursor is converted after interaction with EA into an active enzyme, C' 1 esterase (or C' 1a) in the presence of calcium ions. The complex thus becomes EAC' 1a. The next component of complement to enter the reaction is known as C' 4 which is a β globulin. The complex then becomes EAC' 1a, 4. It seems that C' 4 reacts with a portion of the red cell membrane altered by the enzyme effect of C' 1a. The next step is the interaction of EA C' 1a4 with another β globulin component C' 2. This component is believed to attach to a receptor on C' 4 and is then acted upon by C' 1a to form a new enzyme C' 2a. Six additional complement components are necessary to bring about haemolysis of the complex and in human serum these are known as C' 3, C' 5, C' 6, C' 7, C' 8 and C' 9. Until a few years ago the individual components of this group of β globulins had not been isolated and the activity of the complex was referred to as C' 3 activity. The biochemical events associated with the interaction of these components with the EAC' 1a, 4, 2a complex are thought to be due to an effect on a phospholipid component of the cell membrane but they remain to be elucidated. The result is the production of nearly circular holes 80–100 Å in diameter in the red cell membrane with the resulting lysis of the cell.

Red cell lysis whilst the most intensively studied complement activity is by no means the only role played by the complex. Complement action is of some considerable importance because of its ability to neutralize various types of cell such as human cells or Gram-negative bacteria after they have interacted with antibody. Complement appears to render the bacteria susceptible to lysozyme. Tumour cells for example can survive indefinitely in the presence of antibody but on the addition of complement the cells develop blebs in the membrane, become fragile and lose many of their intracellular constituents leading to death of the cell. Another extremely important role of complement is in the attraction of polymorphonuclear phagocytes to sites of antigen-antibody interaction. This important step in the inflammatory process is known as chemotaxis and appears to depend on the components C' 5, 6 and 7 interacting with the C' 1a, 4, 2, 3 complex. In hypersensitivity states (Chap. 6) complement activation is responsible for the formation of substances known as *anaphylotoxins* three of which are identifiable by MW differences

13

(7,500, 8,500 and 10,000). They arise after C′ 3 and C′ 5 activation and are responsible for bringing about the release of histamine leading to increased vascular permeability and smooth muscle contraction. The formation of the plasma kinins, e.g. bradykinin, which are also active in hypersensitivity states, also appears to depend upon complement activation. Complement components C′ 1–C′ 3 are concerned in promoting phagocytosis and act as opsonins (p. 47).

Normal human serum contains an inhibitor (an α_2-neuramino-glycoprotein) of C′ 1a esterase. This inhibitor may be quantitatively or qualitatively deficient and lead to the condition known as hereditary angioneurotic oedema. The effects are probably due to the formation of anaphylotoxins with the consequent release of histamine. In laboratory practice complement lysis tests have wide and important applications (p. 149).

FURTHER READING

Bacteriological Reviews (1960). Symposium on mechanisms of non-specific resistance to infection, **24,** 1.

van Furth, R. (1970). *Mononuclear Phagocytes*. Oxford & Edinburgh: Blackwell.

Howard, J. G. (1963). Natural immunity. In *Modern Trends in Immunology I*. Ed. Cruickshank, R. London: Butterworth.

Mackaness, G. B. & Blanden, R. V. (1967). Cellular immunity. *Progr. Allergy,* **11,** 89.

Miescher, P. A. & Grabar, P. (1968). Complement. In *Immuno-pathology,* Vol. 5. Basel: Schwabe.

Müller-Eberhard, H. J. (1968). Chemistry and reaction mechanisms of complement. *Adv. Immun.* **8,** 2.

Nelson, D. S. (1968). *Macrophages and Immunity*. Amsterdam: North Holland.

Schur, P. H. & Austen, K. F. (1968). Complement in human disease. *Ann. Rev. Med.* **19,** 1.

Wilson, G. S. & Miles, A. A. (1964). *Topley and Wilson's Principles of Bacteriology and Immunity,* 5th ed. London: Arnold.

Chapter 3

ANTIGENS

Antigens are substances of various chemical types capable of stimulating the immune system of an animal to produce a response specifically directed at the inducing substance and not other unrelated substances. The specificity of the immune response for chemical structures (antigenic determinants) of the antigen molecule is an important characteristic. An antibody directed against an antigenic determinant of a particular molecule will react only with this determinant or another *very similar* structure. Even minor chemical changes in the determinant with the resulting change in shape will markedly alter the ability of the determinant to react with antibody. The term antigen, referring to substances capable of acting as specific stimulants of the immune response or reacting with antibody in an *in vitro* serological test, is used rather loosely by immunologists. Substances which *de novo* are capable themselves of inducing an immune response are sometimes referred to as *immunogens* and are usually large molecules. In contrast, substances (often simple chemicals) incapable alone of inducing an immune response are termed *haptens*. To induce an immune response the hapten requires to be attached to a carrier molecule (usually a serum protein such as albumin). The hapten molecule then acts as a determinant of antigenic specificity and is referred to as an *antigenic determinant*. Immunogens also have antigenic determinants which are simply particular chemical groupings within the macromolecule.

It is important at this point to distinguish clearly between structural specificity of an antigenic determinant and its distribution specificity. For example the ubiquitous nature of the glucose molecule – present in many different types of macromolecule – must be distinguished from its specific chemical structure. An immune response against a glucose determinant in antigen AG would be likely to react also with glucose in antigen

BG provided the two determinants are equally accessible. The antibody directed against the glucose determinant is not as is sometimes thought a non-specific type of antibody but is simply reacting with an identical chemical determinant in another antigen molecule. A typical cross reaction is with pneumococcal polysaccharide type S–V111 which has a tetrasaccharide repeating unit containing cellobiuronic acid alternating with an isomer of lactose. Antisera to such a structure will cross react with oxidized cotton cellulose containing cellobiuronic acid residues. In laboratory serological practice, cross reactions are a common source of difficulty, and cross reactivity is often found between antisera to certain bacterial antigens and antigens present in cells such as erythrocytes. Antigens shared in this way are known as *heterophile antigens* and antisera to these will cross react with cells or fluids of many different species of animal and with various microorganisms. The chemical determinants responsible for this cross reactivity are not known but are presumed to be similar or identical groupings possibly of muco-polysaccharide and lipid nature present in large structural molecules. The best known of the heterophile antigens is the Forssman antigen which is present in the red cells of many species as well as in bacteria such as pneumococci and salmonellae. Another heterophile antigen is found in *E. coli* and human red cells of group B. Another important example is the cross reaction between *Treponema pallidum* and an extract of mammalian heart – cardiolipin. The common shared antigenic structures are phosphatidylglycerols differing only in their fatty acid side groups. Cardiolipin, being more readily available than *Treponema pallidum,* serves as a useful antigen in the serological tests for syphilis (p. 149).

It is common to classify antigens as protein polysaccharides or lipids; this is however an oversimplified view as although many molecules of entirely protein, polysaccharide or lipid nature are antigens it is also not infrequent to find carbohydrate moieties as determinants on protein or lipid macromolecules or peptide units as determinants on polysaccharide macromolecules.

Unfortunately in the present state of knowledge of the antigenic determinants of protein molecules so little information is available about the precise nature of the peptides acting as determinants in different protein macromolecules that immunologists still describe antigens in terms of the whole molecule, e.g. bovine serum albumin (BSA) rather than the individual determinants of specificity within the macromolecule.

Antigenic Determinants

Degradation, chemical modification and synthesis of determinants

The number of determinants (sometimes referred to as its valency) in a molecule like BSA is probably in excess of 18 although only about 6 of these are exposed in the native intact molecule. The other (hidden) determinants can be identified only when the molecule is broken down by, for example, enzyme hydrolysis. Antibody produced in response to injection of the whole molecule appears to be able to react with the fragments produced by hydrolysis, and it therefore appears that the molecule is broken down into similar fragments after injection. This might be brought about by the digestive enzymes in phagocytic cells (p. 10).

Attempts to identify the chemical nature of antigenic determinants have used this type of degradation procedure with some degree of success and some insight has been gained into the size and other features of the determinants. Two other approaches have also been used – chemical modification of known determinants and synthesis of polyamino acid and polysaccharide antigens.

Degradation studies have been carried out on silk fibroin, a linear polypeptide chain of molecular weight between 50,000 and 60,000. The determinant site capable of reacting with antibody appears to consist of between 8 to 12 amino acids (27–44Å) with the C terminal tyrosine making a considerable contribution to the site. The important role of tyrosine is further supported by the finding that the poor antigen gelatin can be made antigenic by the addition of tyrosine in which the native molecule is very deficient. The possibility that tyrosine confers rigidity on the gelatin molecule has been suggested.

The protein coat of tobacco mosiac virus consists of identical subunits (approx. 2000) each with a molecular weight of about 16,500 consisting of 158 amino acids. The antigenic determinant site is present in the chain between position 108 and 112 and unlike fibroin contains no aromatic amino acids. The hydrophobic nature of leucine appears to be an important characteristic of this particular determinant site.

The blood group substances are large molecules consisting of

17

about 75 per cent polysaccharide and 25 per cent polypeptide. Degradation studies have shown that the substances owe their specificity to groups at the end of the carbohydrate chains, for example, A substance specificity is determined by α-N-acetyl-galactosaminoyl – (1–3) – galactose.

A substance which acts as an antigen in one species of animal may not do so in another because it is represented in the tissues or fluids of the second species. This underlines the requirement that an antigen must be a foreign substance to elicit an immune response. For example, it follows that egg albumin whilst an excellent antigen in the rabbit, fails to induce an antibody response in a fowl. The more foreign a substance is to a particular species the more likely it is to be a powerful antigen. A good antigen need not contain different building blocks, e.g. amino acids of a protein, but their arrangement should be such that at least part of the surface of the molecule presents a configuration which is unfamiliar to the animal. Since macromolecules have a three dimensional structure, it is easy to visualize how they could become unfolded by denaturation so as to present new and unique surface arrangements.

Foreignness can be a property which depends on chemical groupings which are entirely unfamiliar to the animal. Arsonic acid, for example, can be introduced by diazotization into a protein molecule. Such a group is known as a *hapten* and acts as the *determinant* of the *antigenic specificity* of the molecule, the protein to which the hapten is attached functioning simply as a *carrier molecule*.

Karl Landsteiner in the early part of this century carried out very extensive studies on the antigenic specificity of such hapten chemical determinants resulting in a new appreciation of how critical and precise was the fit between antibody and an antigenic determinant. Landsteiner's work with, for example, the arsonic acid determinant (AsO_3H_2) showed that changes, even as minor as the replacement in the benzine ring, of the AsO_3H_2 group by a COOH or a SO_3H group (Fig. 2) was sufficient to affect substantially the ability of azo proteins containing the determinant to react with antibody against the unchanged hapten. The influence of changes in shape brought about without the removal or substitution of groups is shown by studies with stereoisomers of macromolecules containing tartaric acid where the antibody to L tartaric acid fails to combine with its isomer D tartaric acid.

Fig. 2 Rabbit antisera to azoproteins containing any of the above acid radicals as antigenic determinants react only with the inducing azoprotein and not with any of the others. Even azoproteins obtained by changing the —COOH of *m*-amino benzoic acid or the —SO$_3$H of metanilic acid to the ortho or para positions do not react with antisera to the original determinant. Methyl and halogen radicals substituted in the benzene ring instead of the acid radicals shown in the figure are less effective as determinants of specificity and considerable cross reactions are found in precipitin tests.

It was concluded from studies of this type (a) that acidic and basic groups are very important in regulating the specificity of an antigenic determinant, (b) that spatial configuration of haptens is important, (c) that terminal groups in an antigen are often important determinants of specificity and (d) that interchange of non-ionic groups of similar size had little effect on specificity of a determinant.

It became clear from studies of this type that a very slight variation in the chemical constitution or even shape of a molecule could substantially affect the ability of antibody to combine with it. Despite this knowledge immunologists even today are still far from understanding the chemical nature of the determinant groups in complex proteins and polysaccharides. Studies by Sela in Israel with synthetic polypeptides show that the surface arrangements of the amino acids in a branched polyamino acid structure are critical as determinants of antigenic specificity (Fig. 3). If the three dimensional structure of a protein is altered by heating or other form of denaturation, it is no longer able to

■ Tyrosine

● Glutamic acid

▨ Poly amino acid backbone

Fig. 3 The amino acids, tyrosine, glutamic acid can convert a non-antigenic polyamino acid branched structure (polyalanine and polylysine) into an antigen provided they are attached to the outer end of the branches (left); if attached at the inner end of the branches (right) the complex is not antigenic.

combine as effectively with antibody to the original native molecule. Enzymes act as antigens and RNAse molecules after oxidation become unfolded and the change in shape prevents the interaction of the molecule with antibody to native RNAse.

Size and physical state

For a substance to be antigenic in its own right without the need to be attached to a carrier molecule requires that it has certain properties which have not yet been fully defined. Amongst these is the fact that high molecular weight materials are better antigens than those of low molecular weight. A substance below a molecular weight of about 5000 is not likely to be a good antigen. This phenomenon may be partly explained by the presence in a larger molecule of repeating antigenic determinant groups, and in a complex molecule of a large variety of potential determinants, one or more being capable of preferentially stimulating an immune response. Large molecular size alone is not sufficient to confer antigenicity on a substance. Synthetic polymers of many types can be built up into large macromolecules and are non-antigenic. The polyamino acid backbone (polyalanine and polylysine) of the molecule shown in Figure 3 is non-antigenic and only becomes capable of inducing an immune response by the addition of further different amino acids. It has been suggested that the lack of antigenicity of synthetic polymers is due to their lack of internal molecular complexity. Thus the antigenicity of naturally occurring macromolecules may be due to their many different low molecular weight constituents giving complexity to the molecule.

The physical state of a protein antigen can affect its antigenicity. The same substance, e.g. the serum protein BSA, in aggregated and aggregate-free form can show wide divergence in ability to stimulate immunity, the aggregated form being strongly antigenic in the rabbit while the aggregate-free form induces a specific state of unresponsiveness (immunological tolerance, p. 50).

Some molecules carry what is sometimes called 'built-in-adjuvanticity' which means that they have the capacity to stimulate the cells of the antibody system in a non-specific manner so that they are able to handle antigen more effectively. Bacterial endotoxin produces this effect as also do *Bordetella pertussis* organisms and these materials can enhance the antigenicity of a weak antigen if administered at the same time. In human immunization the efficacy of the 'triple vaccine', diphtheria, pertussis, tetanus, is partly due to the effect of *B. pertussis* (p. 104). Polysaccharide antigen, for example dextran of molecular weight (MW) 600,000 is a good antigen, whereas a dextran of MW 100,000 is not. There is no obvious reason for this as the two materials are made up of identical building blocks and do not differ as far as the type of antigenic determinant is concerned.

Some low molecular weight chemical substances appear to contradict the need noted above that an antigen be a large molecule. Among these are included picryl chloride, formaldehyde, and drugs such as aspirin, penicillin and sulphonamides. These substances are highly antigenic, particularly if applied to the skin. The reason for this appears to be that such materials form complexes by means of covalent bonds with tissue protein, and the complex of these substances, acting as haptens with tissue protein carrier forms complete antigen. This has important implications in the development of certain types of hypersensitivity states (p. 80).

The ability of an animal to degrade a polysaccharide antigen can affect its immune reactivity to the antigen. Some pneumococcal polysaccharides appear to be resistant to digestion in the mouse and in sufficient dose are able to mop up antibody as it is made, resulting in the absence of detectable antibody in the serum.

FURTHER READING

Barrett, J. T. (1970). *Textbook of Immunology*. London: Kimpton.

Boyd, W. C. (1963). *Fundamentals of Immunology*. London:Inter-science.

Dumonde, D. C. (1965). Tissue specific antigens. *Adv. Immun.* **5,** 30.

Heidelberger, M. (1956). *Lectures in Immunochemistry*. New York: Academic Press.

Kabat, E. A. (1968). *Structural Concepts in Immunology and Immunochemistry*. New York: Holt, Rinehart & Winston.

Landsteiner, K. (1945). *The Specificity of Serological Reactions*. Cambridge, Mass: Harvard University Press.

Sela, M. (1965). Immunological studies with synthetic polypeptides. *Adv. Immun.* **5,** 30.

Chapter 4

ACQUIRED IMMUNITY

Microorganisms which overcome or circumvent the innate non-specific immune mechanisms come up against the host's second line of defence. To give expression to this form of immunity it is necessary that antigens of the invading microorganisms come in contact with cells of the immune system (macrophages and lymphocytes) which leads to the initiation of an immune response specific for the inducing antigen. This response takes two forms which usually develop in parallel.

1. Humoral immunity

The characteristic of this form of immunity is the appearance in the blood of globulins known as antibodies or immuno-globulins. These combine specifically with the antigen which stimulates their production and can lead to some remarkable consequences. For example, the antigen molecules or particles may be clumped, their toxicity may be neutralized, their uptake and subsequent digestion by phagocytes facilitated and cellular antigens that are part of a cell surface such as a red blood cell or bacterium may be lysed.

2. Cell-mediated immunity

Lymphoid cells may be induced by prior exposure to antigen, to react subsequently directly with the inducing antigen and bring about cytotoxic effects as for example on foreign cells from a graft. The precise manner in which these sensitized cells perform this function is not understood. This form of immunity is known as cell-mediated immunity.

General features

It is important to note that the immune response is a physio-logical reaction to the introduction into the body of foreign material, irrespective of whether it is harmful or not. Further, the response may be directed at antigens which are inside micro-organisms and thus inaccessible to the serum proteins so that they perform no protective role. In contrast to innate immune mechanisms which vary greatly between species, the acquired response is little different between species and the main differences that can be detected occur between individuals.

An acquired immune state may be brought about in an individual in two main ways: (1) induced by overt clinical infection, inapparent clinical infection or deliberate artificial immunization. This is termed '*actively acquired immunity*' and contrasts with (2) '*passively acquired immunity*' which is transferred from an actively immunized individual to a non-immune individual by means of blood, serum components or experimentally by lymphoid cells.

Table 2

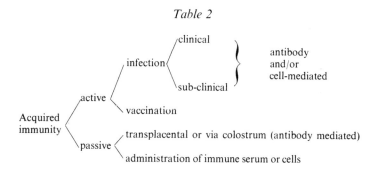

Actively acquired immunity

Actively acquired immunity due to infectious agents fall into two general categories. Some infections, such as diphtheria, whooping cough, smallpox and mumps, usually induce a lifetime immunity. Others such as the common cold, influenza, pneumococcal pneumonia and bacillary dysentery, confer immunity for a shorter time, sometimes for only a few weeks. Failure of the second group of infections to induce lasting immunity is due to various factors, particularly to the fact that different members or strains of the same species of organism may be involved and the acquisition of immunity to one strain does not prevent infection by another strain of the same organism.

Administration of immune sera usually prepared in another species, e.g. the horse, is a therapeutic procedure in diphtheria and in gas gangrene. Anti-tetanic serum is used prophylactically when wounds may be contaminated with tetanus spores. Passive immunity may be conferred on the infant by the passage of maternal antibody across the placenta in some species such as the human and the rabbit, where a particular part of the immuno-globulin polypeptide chain has been found to be necessary for bringing about the transfer process (p. 48). In other species such as the rat and the dog antibodies are also transmitted in the colostrum via the intestine. Other animals, notably the lamb and the calf, receive this form of immunity only by means of the colostrum. Pooled human immunoglobulin is also used as a source of antibody in a number of situations including measles infection and infectious hepatitis, when it is given during the incubation period to modify the attack. Human immuno-globulin is also given to patients with a congenital inability to make antibody globulin (p. 67).

THE IMMUNE RESPONSE

Immunoglobulin Production – the Humoral Antibody Response

The antibody response resulting from exposure to antigenic substances has certain well defined characteristics. After first meeting the antigen there is an interval of about two weeks before antibody can be found in the blood, and during this initial period there is intense activity in the antibody-forming tissues. This can be shown by studies with isotope-labelled precursors of cell com-ponents, for example tritiated thymidine, to show DNA synthesis or carbon-14 labelled amino acids in protein synthesis. Following antigenic stimulation there is a rapid increase in cell proliferation and synthesis of protein in the cells of the lymphoid organs indicated by the incorporation of the labelled materials. In a mouse immunized, for instance, with sheep red blood cells lymphocytes taken from the spleen or lymph nodes can be shown to have synthesized anti-sheep cell antibodies because if sheep red cells are mixed with the spleen or lymph gland cells the red cells aggregate around individual lymphocytes giving a rosette

IMMUNO-CYTO-ADHERENCE — Rosette technique

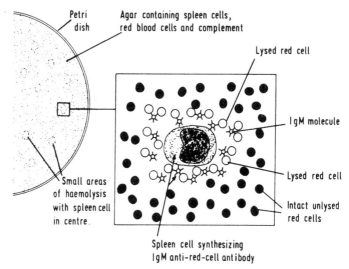

LOCALIZED HAEMOLYSIS IN GEL — Jerne Plaque technique

Fig. 4 Two methods for demonstrating antibody formation by single cells. In the immuno-cyto-adherence test spleen cells from an animal immunized with, for example, sheep red blood cells, are mixed with the red cell antigen and after a period of incubation 'rosettes' are formed as shown. The red cells often completely surround the antibody-producing spleen cell. In the Jerne plaque technique, the spleen cells from the sheep-cell immunized animal are mixed with the red cell antigen in soft agar and when complement (guinea-pig serum) is layered on the surface, lysis of the red cells occurs. This happens because the antibody produced by the spleen cell has diffused into the surrounding agar and coated the red cells. This enables the complement system to be activated with the resulting lysis of the red cell (see p. 12 for description of complement lysis).

appearance when examined microscopically (Fig. 4). The red cells become attached to the surface of lymphocytes by means of antibody located at the cell membrane. The antibody which eventually can be detected in the blood – the so-called **'primary immune response'** does not reach a high level and does not persist unless a second dose of antigen is given (Fig. 5). When this happens, any remaining antibody will be rapidly mopped up by combination with the antigen and this will be reflected by a fall in detectable antibody in the blood; then after only a day or two a remarkable rise in the level of antibody begins and reaches a peak shortly thereafter which can be from 10 to 50 times higher than the primary response. This **'secondary response'** is maintained at a high level falling only slowly over a period of months. The response can be boosted to even higher levels by further injections of antigen until a stage is reached when no further increase occurs. It is important to note that once an animal has responded to an antigen, even although exposed to it on only one occasion, the animal retains a 'memory' of the antigen so that even after an interval of months or years it is able to react by means of a secondary response with a rapid mobilization of antibody-forming cells. Hence vaccination against an infective agent such as smallpox or poliomyelitis virus provides many years of useful protection against infection even though soon after vaccination the level of antibodies falls to a low level, since the memory has been retained.

To obtain a maximum response, the interval between the primary and secondary injections should not be too short and an

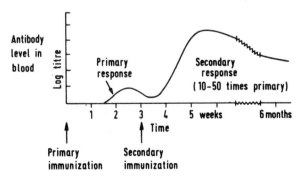

Fig. 5 The antibody response

interval of less than 10 days is likely to reduce the level of the secondary response; subsequent injections should be spaced out to weeks then to months (p. 103). This allows time for the increase in numbers of antibody-forming cells which can be stimulated by subsequent injections.

Some of the host determinants of acquired immunity have already been mentioned. The nature of the antigen, the form in which it is presented, the route of injection and the dose given also have marked effects on the response.

Determinants of Acquired Immunity

Form, dose and route of entry of antigen

The determinants of antigenic specificity have been discussed above (p. 15), as have the effect of molecular weight and the need for foreignness of the antigenic material. It is however possible to enhance the natural ability of an antigen to induce an immune response by altering it or mixing it with another substance (called an adjuvant). A procedure of much practical value is to alter the physical state of the antigen by adsorbing it on to mineral gels such as aluminium hydroxide or phosphate. These alum-precipitated antigens are widely used as immunizing agents for humans. Such particulate forms of antigens seem to be able to initiate antibody production much more effectively than the same antigens in non-particulate form. This effect is not fully understood but may be due to a direct effect of the particulate material on the lymphocyte cell membrane leading to more effective transformation of the cell for antibody formation than can be brought about by antigen in solution. An additional factor which may be important for some types of antigen is that particulate material is more readily phagocytosed by macrophages. These cells have been shown in certain situations to make a contribution by serving as a store of antigen for later release and stimulation of lymphocytes (Fig. 6). It has been suggested that macrophages may also improve the antigenicity of weak antigens by altering them in some way before passing them on to lymphocytes. It is conceivable also that by removing antigen from the circulation they protect the lymphocytes from the effects of excess antigen which would be likely to paralyse the lymphocytes rather than initiate antibody production (p. 50). For a

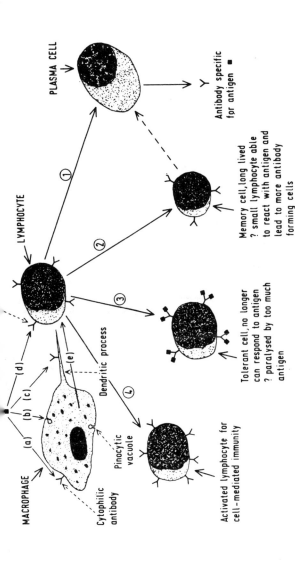

Fig. 6 Antigen can follow four possible routes. (a) Interact with antibody on surface of macrophage and be retained for later transfer to lymphocyte. (b) Enter macrophage by pinocytosis and be either eliminated by digestion or broken into fragments and passed to lymphocyte (e) either along or in combination with macrophage RNA. (c) Interact with antibody on dendritic process of macrophage or perhaps be brought into contact with lymphocyte. (d) Interact directly with antibody receptor on the surface of the lymphocyte or perhaps enter the cell. Four possible consequences are shown. (1) Transformation of lymphocyte to immunoblast-plasma cell leading to antibody production. (2) Production of memory cell to react later with antigen. (3) Tolerant cell after appropriate stimulus which may be excess antigen. (4) Activated lymphocyte for cell-mediated immune reaction.

protein antigen a dose of a few hundred microgrammes is required to stimulate the production of detectable circulating antibody. The increase in antibody response is small in proportion to the increase in dose of antigen given and is approximately proportional to the square root of the increase in antigen administered until an upper limit is reached. An increase above this level can, as indicated above, result in specific paralysis of the antibody-forming tissues. This form of inhibition sometimes referred to as 'immunological tolerance' is specific only for the antigen which brought it about. The lymphoid tissues remain normally responsive to other antigens.

Other methods have been developed to enhance the antibody response, although at present they are used mainly in experimental work. The most important of these consists of the preparation of a water-in-oil emulsion (Fig. 7): an aqueous

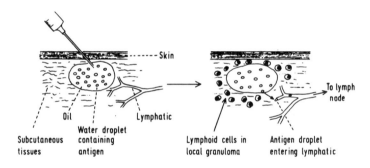

Fig. 7 Water in oil adjuvant (depot forming adjuvant)

solution of antigen is emulsified in a light mineral oil so that tiny drops of antigen solution are dispersed throughout the oil. The emulsion forms a depot of antigen in the subcutaneous tissues from which small quantities of antigen are continually released, sometimes for a year or more. An influenza vaccine in this form has been used successfully in man. New possibilities have been opened up by the development in Edinburgh of a multiple form of emulsion, in which the aqueous solution is first dispersed in oil and the oil is finally dispersed in a water phase. These emulsions are stable and much less viscous and less difficult to inject than the water-in-oil type. An even better response is achieved if killed tubercle bacilli are included in the emulsion; a wax constituent of the bacterial wall is responsible for this effect. The bacterial product appears to stimulate the cells involved in the immune response. Such emulsions are of course suitable for experimental work and are often termed Freund's adjuvants after their originator.

The advantages of these 'adjuvant' methods of immunization are that both the primary and secondary immune response are achieved by only one injection of antigen and that the peak level of antibody is maintained over a long period by the small quantities of antigen released from the depot.

If an antigen is given intravenously most of the antibody is produced by the spleen, and some in the lung and bone marrow; on the other hand, if given subcutaneously or intradermally, the antigen travels via lymphatics to the local lymph nodes where antibody production is initiated. When antigen is given with adjuvants, there is a local accumulation of inflammatory cells, and antibody production occurs in the resulting granulomatous tissue as well as in the draining lymph nodes.

The Cell-mediated Acquired Immune Response

As indicated above, in the immunologically mature individual, contact with an antigen leads not only to the production of circulating antibody, but also to the development of a separate cell-mediated form of response. In both types initial contact with the antigen is necessary and the response is specific for the antigen. Cell-mediated immunity occurs particularly in infections by agents which enter the cells such as viruses, tubercle bacilli and *Brucella* species (p. 48). It can also develop after skin contact with certain simple chemical substances (p. 80). The sequence of steps leading to this form of immunity is essentially no different from that leading to the antibody response but the response is initiated in different areas of the spleen and lymph nodes (white pulp around the central arterioles of the spleen and the para-cortical areas of the lymph nodes); these areas are under the control of the thymus gland (p. 56). A characteristic of these thymus-dependent lymphocytes is that they can be stimulated to differentiate and divide by plant extracts known as phyto-haemagglutinins (PHA) and by certain extracts of micro-organisms such as streptolysin S from streptococci. These

31

substances, sometimes referred to as mitogens, appear to act on the small lymphocytes of all vertebrates so far examined and induce enlargement of the cells, increased synthesis of RNA followed later by DNA synthesis. This process is known as *lymphocyte transformation* and can be brought about in sensitized lymphocytes on subsequent exposure to the sensitizing antigen. Transformation is readily measured *in vitro* by culturing the cells in the presence of labelled precursors of nucleic acids, e.g. ^{14}C thymidine for DNA synthesis or ^{14}C uridine for RNA synthesis. The test can be used to detect sensitization to an antigen and the non-specific plant mitogens are used as a test of the competence of the cell-mediated immune system. Lymphocytes from an individual with, for example, an immune deficiency state (Chap. 5) with thymic aplasia and consequent defective cell-mediated immunity would be unable to transform in the presence of PHA. Transformation of lymphocytes to PHA is reduced in certain virus infections (p. 98).

This type of response is brought about by lymphocytes and is usually recognized by means of a skin test (e.g. intradermal injection) with the antigen that in an individual who has developed a cell-mediated immune response, results in an inflammatory reaction at the injection site. When examined histologically it can be seen that the tissues at the injection site have been infiltrated by mononuclear cells, mainly lymphocytes and a few macrophages.

The part played by these infiltrating lymphocytes in cell-mediated immune reactions was for many years not clearly understood. Recently a group of non-antibody lymphocyte factors or *lymphokines* have been shown to be released from sensitized lymphocytes when they are exposed to antigen. The factors can be recovered in the culture fluid of cells maintained *in vitro* and over the last few years it has been possible partly to purify and assay the lymphokine activity. The best known of these non-antibody factors released by sensitized lymphocytes on contact with antigen has the property of preventing the *in vitro* migration of macrophages on a glass surface. Macrophages can be set up in culture in small capillary tubes and will normally migrate out of the open end of the tube into the culture fluid (Fig. 8). A factor released from lymphocytes exposed to antigen will prevent this migration by causing the macrophages to stick together. This factor is likely to be released also *in vivo* and may

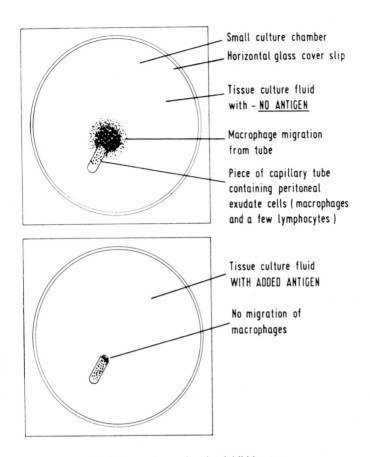

Fig. 8 Macrophage migration inhibition test

be responsible for the accumulation of macrophages in cell-mediated immune reactions (p. 28). A further as yet undefined factor released from sensitized lymphocytes after exposure to antigen causes stimulation and proliferation of normal un-sensitized lymphocytes. This is known as mitogenic factor. Yet another lymphokine has a chemotactic effect on macrophages attracting them to the site of the inflammatory response. A cytotoxic effect, which appears to be due to a lymphokine (lymphotoxin), has also been demonstrated with a damaging effect on a variety of types of cell. A factor which increases capillary permeability (skin reactive factor) can also be shown to be released by sensitized lymphocytes. The overall contribution of these factors in the cell-mediated immune response has not yet been clearly established nor has their chemical identity or mode of action. However it is widely believed that the lymphokines are the main effector mechanism in the cell-mediated responses.

It seems likely that the cell-mediated immune response is involved in protection against various infective agents (p. 97). It may also serve an important physiological role in the normal individual bringing about the elimination of spontaneously arising neoplastic cells which might represent a potential threat to the individual. In support of the existence of such an *immunological surveillance* mechanism (Chap. 11) it has been found that the incidence of tumours is highest at the two extremes of life when the immunological mechanisms are at their least efficient. The cell-mediated immune system is under the influence of the thymus (p. 56) and after thymectomy in mice the incidence of tumours induced by chemical carcinogens and viruses has been found to be significantly higher than in sham-thymectomized controls. The thymus has been found to be absent in certain rare immune deficiency states of children (p. 67). In such conditions there is a deficiency of lymphocytes from the areas of spleen and lymph nodes under thymic control. Cell-mediated immune reactions are absent and there is an inability to deal with virus infections. This type of cell-mediated immune mechanism would be likely to have arisen early in evolution with the development of multicellular organisms and would have additional survival value in that it would also be effective against exogenous parasites.

THE TISSUES INVOLVED IN IMMUNE REACTIONS

The lymphoid tissues which are predominantly engaged in the immune response are the lymph nodes, spleen and bone marrow. Whilst the lung and to a lesser extent the liver can both take part in the immune response, their contribution is much less than that of the other tissues. The large overall contribution of the bone marrow is a reflection of the mass of this tissue throughout the skeleton. However, weight for weight the spleen and lymph nodes by far exceed the capacity for antibody production of the bone marrow. For this reason much effort has been expended in attempting to unravel the way in which the specialized lymphoid organs, the spleen and lymph nodes take up foreign antigens and initiate the immune process.

Gross structure

The lymph nodes of the human are structures of the shape and approximate size of a bean. In smaller animals they are of the the same general structure but correspondingly smaller. The lymph flows from the limbs and organs through the lymph nodes on its way to the main lymphatic vessels of the neck and their union with the veins. The afferent lymphatics enter the capsule of the node (Fig. 9) and the lymph leaves via the efferent lymphatics of the hilium. Trabeculae extend radially into the node

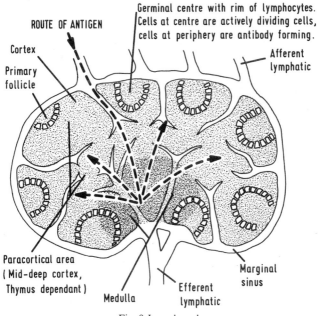

Fig. 9 Lymph node

35

from the capsule passing from the marginal lymph sinus through the cortex to the medulla. The tissue of the gland consists of a meshwork of reticular cells in which large numbers of lymphocytes are embedded. These cells are grouped in nodules or follicles in the cortex and form interconnected cords in the medullary area sometimes called medullary cords. Around each nodule in the cortex is a condensation of reticular cells and macrophages with cytoplasmic extensions or dendritic processes. Macrophages are present throughout the gland, many being found in the medullary area. Plasma cells and their precursors are also found particularly at the cortico-medullary junction.

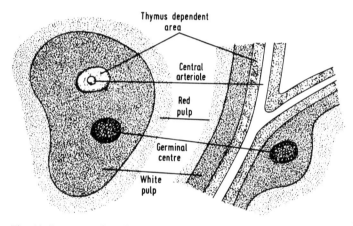

Fig. 10 Structure of Malpighian corpuscle. Transverse section of part of spleen showing area of white pulp related to central arteriole and considered to be thymus-dependent.

The spleen (Fig. 10) like the lymph nodes is enclosed by a capsule and divided by trabeculae into communicating compartments. The tissue consists of (a) the white pulp – around the branches of the splenic artery which are surrounded by periarterial lymphatic sheaths and lymphatic nodules or Malpighian bodies, and (b) the red pulp – splenic sinuses and splenic cords, the latter making up bands of tissue, reticulum cells, erythrocytes, lymphocytes and granulocytes – lying between the sinuses which are themselves lined by 'sinus-lining cells' held together by a network of reticular fibres. The blood leaves the white pulp via capillaries and enters the red pulp passing into the sinuses and is collected up into venules and veins leaving by the splenic vein. The precise details of the blood circulation in the spleen are not yet fully elucidated, but particulate material and cells can clearly pass through the walls of splenic vessels or be discharged directly into the splenic tissue (p. 62). It can thus be seen that the lymph nodes and spleen can be regarded as a complex organization of three types of cell involved in the initiation of the immune reaction – lymphocytes, plasma cells and phagocytic cells of the reticulo-endothelial system.

This account of the structure and histological detail of the spleen and lymph nodes must not obscure the fact that many of the cells in these organs are part of a mobile population circulating between the blood and lymphoid tissues (p. 61).

Development

The lymphoid tissues responsible for humoral antibody production are associated developmentally with the gut and consist of lymphocytes and plasma cells of the lymph node and spleen. The lymphoid tissues responsible for cell-mediated immune reactivity are associated with the thymus (see pp. 56–61 for further discussion on this subject). In both the spleen and lymph nodes there are areas of lymphoid tissues under the influence of the thymus – the so-called thymus-dependent areas (Fig. 10) – lying adjacent to the central arterioles in the spleen and the post-capillary venules in the medulla of the lymph node. After experimental neonatal thymectomy these areas do not develop properly and cell-mediated immune reactions are absent. There is a rare human condition (Di George's syndrome, p. 67) where this occurs in the absence of thymus function. Histological examination of the spleen and lymph nodes shows that the areas described are deficient in cells.

In the humoral immune response, immunoglobulins are secreted into the blood by lymphoid cells – predominantly plasma cells situated in the spleen and lymph nodes. In contrast the cell-mediated response when it occurs peripherally (e.g. in the skin) is effected by migration of the stimulated cells themselves from the lymphoid tissue via the efferent lymphatics to the blood stream, which some of the cells leave through the capillary endothelium to pass into the tissue fluids where they are ready to interact with foreign antigenic material. These cells are then collected by the afferent lymphatics and recirculate. Organized lymphoid tissues are absent in invertebrates and the most primitive of the vertebrates, the hag fish. This system develops late in phylogeny and the first traces appear in the lamprey. Both these primitive vertebrates are however able to show a limited degree of adaptive immunity. Their serum contains a primitive form of immunoglobulin which has since become considerably diversified. The precursors of the early immuno-globulins are likely to have arisen in the prevertebrate era although as yet there is no direct evidence for this. It has been suggested that they may have arisen from receptors on the surface of phagocytes which enable the cells to distinguish foreign material from self. It seems possible that such receptors could have the molecular properties of the combining site of an antibody molecule. The complement system appeared some time later in evolution and is developed in the jawed vertebrate, the paddle fish. With increasing structural complexity of animal species the immune reaction has become more diversified and effective. However once components of the immune system appear in evolution they are maintained with a remarkable constancy both at the molecular and functional level.

In the human, lymphoid tissue appears first in the thymus at about eight weeks' gestation. Peyer's patches are distinguishable by the fifth month and immunoglobulin secreting cells appear in the spleen and lymph nodes at about 20 weeks. From this period onwards both IgM and IgG globulins (p. 42) are synthes-ized by the foetus with IgM predominating. At birth the infant has a blood concentration of IgG comparable to, or sometimes higher than, that of maternal serum having received IgG but not IgM via the placenta from the mother (p. 48). The rate of synthesis of IgM in the infant increases rapidly within the first few days of life but does not reach adult levels until about a year. This compares with the much slower rise in IgG and IgA globulins which do not reach adult levels until between the sixth and seventh years of life. Cell-mediated immune reactions can be stimulated at birth but these reactions (e.g. homograft rejection) may not be as powerful as in the adult, although the evidence for this is rather scanty.

THE IMMUNOGLOBULINS

Enormous advances have been made in the last decade in knowledge of the chemical structure of immunoglobulins and the relationship of the structure to the biological activities of the molecule. These have enabled immunologists to agree internationally on a nomenclature which distinguishes a number of different classes of immunoglobulin on structural rather than functional characteristics. It was the practice to refer to an antibody as an agglutinin, a neutralizing or a precipitating antibody when it was not realized that each of these activities could be exhibited by a chemically heterogeneous population of molecules and could be shared by the same molecule. Other classifications were dependent on the behaviour of the molecules in electrophoresis which did little more than split the population up into still heterogeneous groups of proteins differing in their overall charge and molecular size.

Methods have been developed in America for the fragmentation of the immunoglobulin molecule by chemical cleavage in Edelman's laboratory, and by pepsin digestion by Nisonoff. Porter in Britain, was the first to achieve cleavage with retention of biological activity of the fragments using pepsin digestion. These studies gave impetus to the work which now has enabled immunologists to distinguish five main classes of immunoglobulin each based on a similar polypeptide chain structure consisting of two pairs of 'heavy' and 'light' chains joined by disulphide bonds sometimes occurring as multiples of this basic unit.

It is considered that the molecule is based on a 12-unit structure, each unit consisting of a polypeptide chain with 110 amino acids of MW 12,000. Each light chain of MW 25,000 consists of two of the basic units and each heavy chain four basic units. Heterogeneity of immunoglobulin structure occurs within this general framework with some of the basic units being affected more than others. Figure 11 shows a tentative view of how the molecule may have evolved from the basic unit, perhaps arising as a receptor on a phagocytic cell. The evolutionary advantage provided by antibody-like molecules has ensured their maintenance and diversification over hundreds of millions of years. A picture of the immunoglobulin molecule has been built up

Fig. 11 Possible evolution of the immunoglobulin molecule.

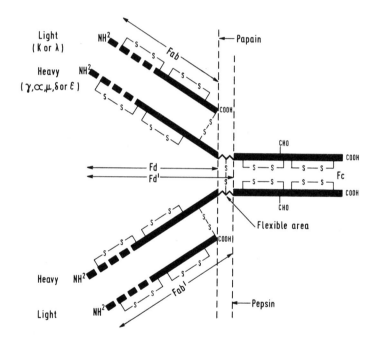

Fig. 12 Diagrammatic view of structural arrangements of polypeptide chains of immunoglobulin molecule. The chains are held together by three disulphide bonds. Papain and pepsin split the molecule on each side of the disulphide bond holding the two heavy chains together, leaving an Fc fragment (crystallizable) and Fd or Fd¹ parts of the heavy chains with attached light chains – the whole making Fab or Fab¹ (or antigen binding) fragments. The N terminal ends of the light and heavy chains have variable sequences of amino acids as shown by the broken line. There are also a number of intra-chain disulphide bonds which influence the shape of individual chains.

and is represented in Figure 12. The general arrangement has been confirmed by electron microscopy.

On the basis of marked antigenic differences in the heavy chains it has been possible to define five classes of human

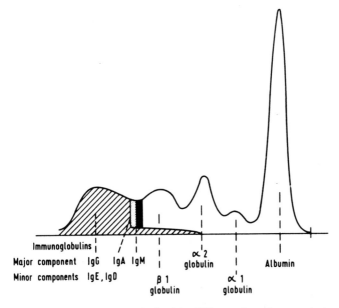

Fig. 13 Electrophoretogram obtained by UV scanning of paper electrophoresis strip and showing diagrammatically the main components of human serum and the immunoglobulin classes.

immunoglobulin, using the technique of immunoelectrophoresis. These are referred to as IgG, IgM, IgA, IgE and IgD (Table 3) (Fig. 13).

Immunoglobulin G or IgG

This is the major immunoglobulin component of serum making up 75 per cent of the total and having a molecular weight of 160,000 in the human. The molecule has two antigen-binding sites as shown in Figure 12 on what are termed the Fab portions of the molecule and involving part of both the heavy and light

Table 3 Human immunoglobulins
(Levels vary widely, males tend to have slightly lower levels of IgG and IgM but higher IgA)

Immunoglobulin class	Serum concentration mg/100 ml	Molecular weight	Half life days	Light chains	Heavy chains	Characteristic properties
IgG	900–1800	160,000	18–23	K and L	γ	Precipitins Antitoxins Complement fixation Late antibody
IgA	156–294	160,000 and polymers	5–6.5	K and L	α	Surface protection
IgM	67–145	960,000	5	K and L	μ	Agglutinins Opsonins Lysins, complement fixation Early antibody
IgD	0.3–40	184,000	2.8	K and L	δ	Not known
IgE	0.0001–0.0007	200,000	?	K and L	ε	Reaginic antibody

chains. The amino acid sequences have been worked out in whole or part for a small number of light and heavy chains in various species, using myeloma proteins which are present as a homogeneous population in the serum of individuals with plasma cell tumours in sufficient quantity to enable studies of this type to be made. The light chains can be shown to consist of two parts joined together, one with a constant sequence of amino acids at the C terminal end of the chain common to the light chains of the species under study, and the other at the N terminal end in which variation occurs in the sequence of the 107 amino acids differing between one myeloma and another, being similar only within a particular myeloma. Up to 50 per cent of the positions in the N terminal portion have been found to be variable. This leads to an enormous number of different permutations of sequence and thus in antibody specificity. Similar variation has been found in rather more limited studies of the N terminal end of the heavy chain. The variable portions of the light and heavy chains are contained in the Fab portion of the molecule and it is in this variable portion of the chain that the antigen-binding site is present. No species specific amino acid residues have so far been found in the variable portion and this suggests that during embryogenesis a single gene controls the development of the entire range of variability in the light chains. This gene probably arose early in evolution and the survival value associated with diversification of the antigen-binding site has ensured its maintenance since then. The light chains are of two distinct types known as K or L (κ or λ) chains. In any one individual, both K and L chains are produced but they are not found together in the same immunoglobulin molecule. K and L chains are present in a ratio of about 2:1 in any one individual. Two intra-chain disulphide bonds (Fig. 12) occur in almost exactly the same position in both K and L chains and both chains have cysteine as the terminal amino acid at the carboxyl end. This serves for the attachment to the heavy chains. These facts suggest a common genetic origin of K and L chains which although they have diverged during evolution have retained many common structural characteristics. The heavy chains are however specific for each class; in the human IgG molecule the heavy chain or γ chain exists in four different forms, IgG1, IgG2, IgG3 and IgG4, which can be distinguished by specific antisera able to detect differences in the Fc fragment of the heavy chains.

43

Sixty-five per cent of the IgG molecules in human serum are of the IgG1 subgroup, 23 per cent of the IgG2 and 8 per cent and 4 per cent IgG3 and 4.

Allotypes or Gm and Inv factors of immunoglobulin have been detected. The antigenic groupings determining the Gm group are present only in the γ chains of the IgG molecule whereas the Inv factors are present in the light chains of each of the major immunoglobulin classes. Twenty-six genetically determined allotypes have been described. These globulin differences between individuals can be compared to the blood groups but instead of involving antigenic differences in the red cell surface they depend on antigenic differences in the light and heavy chains of the immunoglobulin molecule.

IgM, IgA and IgD

Like IgG globulin each of these classes of immunoglobulin in man has been found to contain K and L light chains. The heavy chains on the other hand are unique for each of these types of immunoglobulin, IgM containing μ chains, IgA α chains and IgD δ chains and it is these differences which enable them to be distinguished one from another. The Gm factors found in the Fc

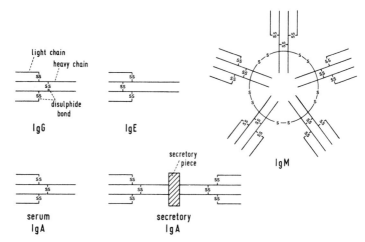

Fig. 14 Diagrammatic view of molecular structure of different immunoglobulin classes.

region of IgG have been found to be absent from a number of IgM and IgA globulins. IgM globulin with a molecular weight of about 900,000 can be split by reduction of disulphide bonds into five subunits. These subunits have a molecular weight of 180,000 and are believed like IgG to have two heavy and two light chains.

Until recently most studies on the number of antigen-binding sites of IgM antibody showed that the molecule had only five binding sites despite the fact that theoretically 10 were present. Both human and rabbit IgM however have now been shown to have the 10 sites and it is believed that the two binding sites on each are unable to combine with antigen with similar efficiency thus making it difficult to demonstrate all 10 sites. The molecular structure of some of these immunoglobulins is shown in Figure 14.

Structure and Function of Immunoglobulin

Knowledge gained from the structural studies discussed above has helped towards an understanding of the biological activities of the immunoglobulin molecule and it is now possible to pinpoint areas of the molecule responsible for different activities. The areas of the light and heavy chains (Fab portion) containing the variable sequences are the site of that part of the molecule with the capacity to combine with antigen. The heavy chain component (Fd portion) seems in some studies to contain as much as 85 per cent of the antigen-binding ability although this is not always so. The light chain component although usually inactive alone seems to act together with the heavy chain to form a stable antigen-binding site.

Complement activation and agglutination

The Fc portion of the molecule appears in IgG molecules to be the major component responsible for activating the complement system, although this does not occur unless two or more molecules of IgG are brought into close apposition. It is not certain exactly what changes in molecular configuration or other effects take place when the molecules come close together but isolated Fc fragments do not activate complement and will do so

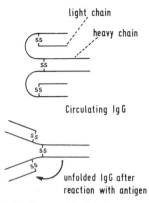

light chain

heavy chain

Circulating Ig G

unfolded IgG after
reaction with antigen

Fig. 15 Possible molecular forms of IgG before and after combination with antigen (see text).

only if aggregated first. One suggestion is shown in Figure 15 in which IgG that has not combined with antigen is represented as folded so that the Fc portion is partly hidden. On combination with antigen the molecule springs open at the hinge region thus exposing the Fc portion which can then activate complement. It has been calculated that a single IgM molecule attached to a red cell by its multiple combining sites can bring about lysis whereas 1000 IgG molecules are required for the same effect. Humphrey and Dourmashkin who came to these conclusions assume that as two IgG molecules must come together for complement activation, a large number of IgG molecules would be required for this to occur as the antigenic determinants are spread evenly over the surface of the red cell. Agglutination is brought about by the linking of particulate antigens such as red cells or bacteria by the two Fab fragments of the immunoglobulin molecule. As might be expected from knowledge of the structure of the IgM molecule its five combining sites make it a very efficient agglutinating antibody molecule and rabbit IgM anti-bacterial antibody is known to be 22 times as active as IgG antibody (mol/mol) in bringing about bacterial agglutination. Because of its large molecular size IgM is largely confined to the blood stream and probably plays an important role in protection. Deficiency of IgM is often associated with susceptibility to septicaemia. IgG antibodies on the other hand are more effective than IgM antibodies at neutralizing diphtheria toxin, lysozyme

46

or viruses such as poliovirus. Whilst some of this activity was present in isolated Fab fragments the evidence from virus neutralization indicates that the Fc fragment may assist the Fab fragments in neutralization of virus infectivity. The molecular basis for such effects has yet to be elucidated.

Tissue fixation and opsonization

The ability of immunoglobulin to attach to tissue cells appears to be a well marked feature of the IgE class of immunoglobulin responsible in humans for various forms of hypersensitivity reaction (p. 72) and may be dependent on the activity of the Fc portion of the molecule. This is suggested by studies of the ability of immunoglobulin fragments to adhere to guinea-pig skin and produce a particular form of hypersensitivity reaction that is known as passive cutaneous anaphylaxis. Immunoglobulin antibody specific for particulate antigens such as bacteria plays a valuable role by coating the surface and making the antigen more susceptible to phagocytosis. These are known as opsonizing antibodies and IgM antibodies perform this role particularly efficiently. In the rabbit it has been shown that IgM anti-salmonella antibodies are some 500–1000 times more effective than IgG antibodies as opsonizing agents. How opsonization is brought about is not clear; it is possible that antibody may alter the surface properties, such as the surface charge of a particulate antigen and thus perhaps electrostatic repulsion between phago-cyte and antigen. It is also conceivable that the Fc fragments of the antibody might have an affinity for the surface of the macrophage and thus link the particulate antigen (attached by means of the antibody combining sites) to the macrophage (attached by the Fc fragment). In support of this possibility, antibody with the ability to attach to macrophages by means of the Fc fragment has been described in the guinea-pig and is known as cytophilic antibody. Antigen-antibody complexes appear to be localized in the lymphoid follicles of lymph glands due to the activity of the Fc portion of the immunoglobulin molecule.

Selective transport

The newborn animal emerging from an environment where it has been sheltered from antigenic stimuli is protected by maternal immunoglobulins transmitted from the mother. These antibodies often reach a level higher than in the mother and persist longer in the circulation of the young animal than they would do in the adult. This transferred passive immunity tides the infant over the period until its own immunological system begins to mature.

In humans, IgG globulins can pass through the placenta and reach the foetal circulation; this is not a simple filtration process, but is due to selective transfer of the molecules involving a part of the Fc fragment of IgG heavy chains. This property is a feature only of the γ heavy chain of IgG and has not been found in the μ and α chains of IgM and IgA. This mechanism seems to be limited to primates whilst in ruminants maternal immunoglobulins from the colostrum reach the foetus through the intestinal epithelium.

Another selective transport mechanism is found with IgA globulins which are selectively secreted into saliva and respiratory and intestinal mucous secretions as well as into the colostrum. The IgA found in these secretions is manufactured locally and has an attached secretory or transport piece not found in serum IgA and it seems likely that it is added to the molecule during its passage into the mucous secretions from the lamina propria, underlying the mucous membrane of the gut and respiratory tract. At the same time as the secretory piece is added the monomeric IgA molecule is turned into a dimer. Salivary and colostral IgA, probably because of the attached secretory piece, appears to be relatively resistant to digestion by proteolytic enzyme lysozyme (p. 8) to digest the mucopolysaccharides of clearly be an advantage in allowing this immunoglobulin to remain active and able to perform a protective role in the intestinal tract. The dimer form of IgA gains the ability to fix complement and after attaching to Gram-negative organisms the activation of the complement system by the IgA allows the enzyme lysozyme (p.   ) to digest the mucopolysaccharides of the microorganism's cell wall. The monomeric form of IgA can also pass from the lamina propria to the blood stream via the lymphatics and gut infections can lead to increased serum IgA levels. Much effort is being expended by laboratory workers in studying the role of IgA as a protective mechanism at the mucous surface and the possible future use of vaccines designed to stimulate this form of antibody response may be of considerable value.

THE CELLS CONCERNED IN ANTIBODY PRODUCTION

Antigen localization and contact with macrophages and lymphocytes

A simplified picture of the cellular mechanisms leading to antibody formation is that antibodies of different specificities are made by different families or clones of cells, each family being genetically programmed to make antibody of only one specificity. There is evidence to show that the cells carry at least part of the molecule of their particular antibody exposed on the cell membrane as a receptor for antigen. Thus when an antigen is injected into the body and comes in contact with lymphoid cells it combines with those exposed antibody receptors which are best able to fit the determinant groups of the antigen molecule.

The way this is brought about can be seen when isotope-labelled antigen is injected into an animal when it is first rapidly localized in the sinus-lining macrophages in the marginal zone around the Malpighian bodies in the spleen or the medullary macrophages of the lymph nodes (Fig. 9), depending on the route of injection (p. 31). After this localization, plasma cell precursors (probably small lymphocytes) at the cortico-medullary junction of the lymph nodes are triggered to proliferate and differentiate into antibody-producing cells; exactly how this triggering mechanism works is not yet understood. One possibility is that after partial degradation in the macrophage, antigenic fragments are passed on to the lymphocytes. It is also possible that some antigens can react directly with the lymphocytes themselves (p. 29). This stimulation and proliferation lead to the development of lymphoid follicles, which are localized collections of active lymphoid cells taking part in the primary immune response. Subsequent contact with antigen now results in a rather different pattern of localization influenced by the presence of secreted antibody to the antigen; antigen whilst still taken up by medullary macrophages is also localized on the surface of dendritic macrophages (macrophages with cytoplasmic extensions) which interdigitate with each other and with the lymphoid cells of the lymphoid follicles or Malpighian bodies. This localization seems to depend on antibody at the surface of the macrophage. Lymphocytes themselves may also come directly in contact with antigen. They can be shown to have at

49

least portions of the immunoglobulin molecule on their surface because they can readily be stimulated to respond by transformation, to contact with antibodies directed at various parts of the immunoglobulin molecule. It seems likely that an individual lymphocyte is coated with fragments, or perhaps whole molecules, of each of the immunoglobulin classes. The specificity of these surface immunoglobulins is thought to be determined by the genetic constitution of the particular lymphocyte. The presence of the antigen at the surface of the lymphocyte is to induce it to transform and proliferate to produce active antibody-producing cells. The mechanism whereby this change is brought about is not clear but certain antigens, e.g. bacterial flagella and keyhole limpet haemocyanin, appear to be readily able to bring about lymphocyte transformation leading to antibody production. Other antigens appear to be less active and require to be taken into macrophages and processed in such a way that they can then influence lymphocytes. Some antigen may be retained at the surface of macrophages where it serves as a depot of antigen for the maintenance of the immune response. It is also possible that some antigen retained within the macrophage will function in this way although antigen can also be catabolized within the macrophage and later eliminated from the body as breakdown products.

Another possible result of the interaction of certain types of antigen, e.g. soluble protein antigens, with the surface of lymphocytes is that the cell is prevented in some way from transforming for antibody production and is thus functionally eliminated from further participation in the immune response. This phenomenon is known as **immune tolerance** and is specific for the inducing antigen, and the term is used by immunologists to indicate a state in which the individual is unable to respond to a specific antigen or hapten. The phenomenon whilst recognized in 1924 by Glenny and Hopkins was first studied experimentally, by Medawar and his colleagues, in mice injected neonatally with cells from another strain of mice (i.e. containing transplantation antigens) (p. 83). The injected mice were later able to accept grafts from the strain of mice which had donated the original injected cells. It has since been found that tolerance to a large variety of antigens can be readily induced when the antigens are injected neonatally. Tolerance can also be induced in the adult provided more antigen is given to take into account the maturity of the lymphoid system, the larger size of the lymphoid organs and thus the more cells to paralyse. A notable advance was made in this field when Mitchison using serum protein antigens showed that there was another form of tolerance inducible by very small doses of antigen. This was termed low zone tolerance in contrast to the high zone tolerance previously described. Doses between these two levels were found to immunize. Other workers have confirmed these findings with different types of antigen. Despite considerable effort on the part of laboratory workers immunologists do not as yet understand the mechanisms underlying tolerance induction but the phenomenon has important implications, particularly in its low zone form, for transplantation immunology (p. 87).

Immunoglobulin synthesis

After these initial changes of transformation of lymphocytes have been set in motion, the actual *synthesis* of large amounts of immunoglobulin takes place. Two types of cell have been shown to be engaged in this process: (1) cells of the plasmocytic series and (2) cells of the lymphocytic series (small, medium and large lymphocytes). Of these two types the plasma cell line makes the largest contribution to immunoglobulin production and when single cells from immunized animals are examined in microdrops it can be shown that two-thirds of the *antibody producing cells* are of this type (Fig. 16). An important characteristic of any cell making immunoglobulin is the presence of a rough endoplasmic reticulum (formed by the attachment of protein-synthesizing polyribosomes to the convoluted endoplasmic reticulum membrane). The lymphocytes contain less of this than do plasma cells. It has been shown by a number of techniques that the immunoglobulin is localized in the spaces of the endoplasmic reticulum where it sometimes forms distinct aggregates termed Russell bodies.

In the spleen the cells engaged in antibody production tend to be found in the red pulp, and in the lymph glands in germinal centres of the cortex.

Individual immunoglobulin-producing cells appear to be able to synthesize the whole molecule, both heavy and light polypeptide chains (p. 43). It has also been found that the individual cells make only one class of immunoglobulin and that the light

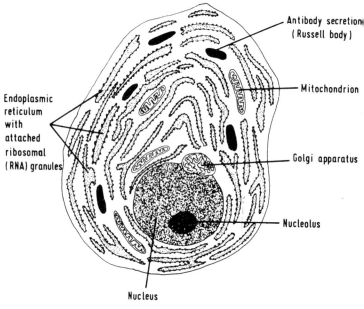

Fig. 16 Plasma cell

chains are restricted to only one of the two types (K and L, p.
43). It is very unusual to find an immunoglobulin secreting cell
synthesizing more than one class of immunoglobulin and it seems
likely that the individual classes found during an immune
response are made by different groups of cells. It is conceivable
that the cell which receives the initial stimulus for transformation
to an antibody-producing cell is initially multipotent as far as its
ability to make different classes of immunoglobulin is concerned.
Once it has become committed, depending perhaps on the nature
of the stimulus, its abilities are then restricted to producing one
class of immunoglobulin.

THE CELLULAR PROCESSES
INVOLVED IN ANTIBODY FORMATION

Learning and memory

The outstanding feature underlying these mechanisms is that
the immune response is a *learning process* at the cellular level.

After initial contact with an antigen the cells of the immune system retain a memory which can be evoked on subsequent contact with the antigen, and furthermore, like other learning processes, the immune system becomes increasingly skilled with continued experience of a particular antigen. The antibody which is synthesized becomes increasingly more effective in binding with antigens, as those cells which are best able to produce a 'good fitting' (avid) antibody molecule are selected from the population of antibody-forming cells. At the same time increasing numbers of committed cells are added to the immune system on repeated contact with antigen and the magnitude of the response is increased (p. 27). This increase in quantity and avidity of antibody can lead for example to increased efficiency in neutralizing an infective agent or its toxic products so that a well immunized animal would be able to withstand a dose of the agent which might be lethal to a poorly immunized animal.

There is at present no satisfactory explanation of the cellular mechanisms which lead to the evocation of either the antibody response or the cell-mediated immune response. This state of affairs is not due to lack of speculation and experimentation, since in the last few years much effort has been directed at solving these problems.

Theories of antibody production

Two main theories have evolved which account for antibody synthesis and are referred to as *directive* and *selective* theories.

Directive theory

The *directive* theory was formulated by Haurowitz, Mudd and Alexander in the early 1930's and later modified by Pauling. The antigen is visualized as a mould or template which can enter any immunoglobulin producing cell and cause the pattern of amino acids laid down to be modified so that it will fit the template, resulting in the synthesis of a molecule with a spatial configuration complementary to that of the antigen molecule. To account for the continued production of antibody it is assumed that the antigen, or part of it, remains in the cell to direct future antibody production. Alternatively, it is proposed that the antigen modifies the genetic information in the DNA of the cell so that it and its daughter cells continue to produce the specific immunoglobulin.

Selective theory

In contrast, the *selective* theory proposes that antigen selects, from the population of cells capable of making antibody, only those few cells that already have the inherent ability to make an immunoglobulin specific for the antigen, the antigen serving simply as a trigger on reacting as suggested above with antibody receptor sites at the lymphocyte cell membrane. *The clonal selection theory* of Burnet is the best known of the selective theories and was formulated and modified over the years to take account of the hitherto unexplained phenomenon of recognition by the normal individual of tissue antigens as part of self and distinguishing these from foreign non-self antigens. Such an explanation became necessary with the description of human diseases where self recognition breaks down and self antigen is treated as if it were foreign antigen – resulting in so-called 'autoimmune disease' (p. 106). The theory proposes that the cells of the antibody-forming system have arisen by random mutation resulting in the emergence of small numbers of cells or clones of cells differentiated so as to be capable of producing one or a very small number of specific antibodies. Contact by such differentiated cells during foetal life before the cells have reached maturity, with self or foreign antigenic material, would lead to suppression rather than stimulation of antibody formation against the particular antigen concerned – immune tolerance. That this could occur was illustrated by the experiments of Medawar and his colleagues on mice which could be induced to accept potentially incompatible skin grafts by pretreatment during neonatal life with the appropriate 'transplantation antigen'. These studies were the forerunner of much further work in this field and it has now been shown that tolerance can also be induced even in adult animals if antigen is given in suitable doses and in an appropriate manner. However it is more difficult to do this in the adult, the immature immune system of the neonatal animal being more susceptible. X-irradiation of an adult is frequently used as an aid in tolerance induction.

Burnet has since suggested that the initial contact with self antigens leading to the elimination of 'self-reactive clones' or 'forbidden clones', may take place in the thymus, this organ acting as a *censor* of the lymphoid cells. This idea is supported by the very rapid turnover of lymphocytes in that organ and by the emergence of self-reactive antibody-producing cells in the absence of the thymus. The view is held by some immunologists that the ageing process may in part be due to a failure in these proposed controlling mechanisms, i.e. a gradual loss of efficiency of the censorship role of the thymus associated with its atrophy later in life.

Implications and variations of theories

The theory outlined above suggests that early contact with self antigens leads to the individual developing an immune system which is suppressed or is tolerant towards self antigens. The unblocking of a cell inherently capable of producing antibody against self antigen would explain auto-antibody formation (p. 108). It is for this aspect of immunity in particular that the clonal selection theory provides a more plausible explanation than the directive theory which requires that all antibody-forming cells are blocked by every self antigen rather than only those cells capable of responding specifically to each antigen concerned. The other main characteristics of antibody formation – the specificity of antibody for antigen and the differences between the primary and secondary responses – can be explained equally well by either theory; the clonal selection theory is however the most complete attempt so far to take into account all the known facts of antibody production. A number of variations of Burnet's original selective hypothesis have been proposed in the last few years but all maintain the assumption that the cell is already programmed to produce a specific antibody. It has been postulated, for example, that each potentially immunologically competent cell carries its chromosomal DNA genes for a large variety of different types of antibody and is thus capable of responding to many antigens. An alternative proposal is that all antibody-producing cells may initially make identical immuno-globulins but during the lifetime of the individual variability of amino acid sequence appears due to crossing over during mitosis of the nucleotides responsible for coding the amino acid sequence of the Fab portion of the molecule. There is a clear survival value in such a variation producing mechanism resulting in the

55

production of immunoglobulins capable of reacting with a wide range of environmental antigens. Similarly there is survival value in the maintenance of those parts of the gene carrying the nucleotide sequences for the constant parts of the immunoglobulin molecule which maintain its structural integrity.

THE ROLE OF THE THYMUS IN IMMUNE REACTIVITY

Development and structure

The thymus in mammals arises from the endoderm of the third and fourth brachial clefts and is the tissue in which lymphocytes can first be recognized. The thymus gland increases in size until puberty and then slowly atrophies although it is still readily recognizable in the adult. The cells of the thymus are of three main types: *thymocytes* morphologically similar to blood lymphocytes, *phagocytic reticulum cells* and *reticular epithelial cells*. The macroscopic structure of the organ is like that of other lymphoid organs in general organization, with a central medulla containing a high proportion of reticular cells and a peripheral cortex containing the thymocytes with some surrounding reticular cells. Unlike the spleen and lymph nodes there are no germinal centres and no plasma cells. Thus under normal physiological conditions the thymus cells do not make antibody. Plasma cells will appear only if antigen is injected directly into the organ. Hassall's corpuscles are a feature peculiar to the medulla of the thymus and consist of groups of reticular epithelial cells sometimes flattened and concentrically arranged around a central core of nuclear debris.

Cell turnover and humoral factor

The thymus can be shown, by tritiated thymidine incorporation studies, to be actively engaged in lymphopoiesis, there being a higher proportion of primitive actively dividing lymphoid cells than in any other lymphoid tissue such as the spleen or lymph nodes, and with a correspondingly high mitotic rate. Evidence suggests that the stimulus for thymocytes to divide arises in some way from the reticular epithelial cells. The primitive cells in the thymus are slowly replaced during life by cells derived from the bone marrow that migrate via the blood stream into the thymus. A small proportion of these cells leave the thymus and find their way to the peripheral lymphoid tissues.

If the thymus is removed during the neonatal period, it is possible to find lymphocyte-deficient areas in the white pulp of the spleen around the central arterioles and in the paracortical area of the lymph nodes. These areas have been termed the 'thymus-dependent' areas of the lymphoid tissues. Associated with this localized deficiency of lymphocytes, neonatally thymectomized animals also have considerably impaired cell-mediated immune effector mechanisms affecting graft rejection and other forms of cell-mediated immunity such as delayed hypersensitivity reactions; humoral immune reactivity is much less markedly affected.

Studies in mice of cell turnover in the adult thymus show that the thymic population of lymphocytes is replaced every three or four days but that the great majority of cells never leave the organ and die there. The reasons for this intense lymphopoiesis is unknown. In the adult it seems that the thymus is necessary for repopulation of lymphoid tissues depleted by X-irradiation or other methods. However studies with chromosome markers have shown that the new cells are not derived directly from the thymus but are lymphoid cells from elsewhere in the body, probably from the bone marrow. The role of the thymus in this situation appears to be the production not of thymus-derived cells but of a humoral factor which restores immunological reactivity to remaining lymphoid cells. This was strongly suggested by experiments in which thymus implants in millipore diffusion chambers were placed in the peritoneal cavity of thymectomized mice. Immunological capacity was restored to the recipients, which recovered the ability to reject skin grafts, although the chambers were impermeable to cells and were on later recovery shown to contain only reticular epithelial and reticulum cells and no lymphocytes. It is worth noting at this point that the hormonal factor produced by the thymus is not the only hormonal influence acting on the lymphoid tissues. Growth hormone increases thymus weight and thyroid hormone increases the weight of the lymphoid tissues and the size of the immune response. Adrenalectomy also increases the weight of the lymphoid tissues, and glucocorticoids, oestrogens and androgens decrease its weight. After neonatal thymectomy acidophilic growth hormone producing cells of the anterior pituitary appear to lose their granules suggesting an increased demand for output of hormone by the cells in the absence of the thymus. Interference with the production of anterior pituitary hormones in mice by means of specific antisera results in lymphocyte depletion in both thymus and spleen. All these observations indicate the close relationship between endocrinological function, immunological maturation and expression of immune capacity.

The essential functions of the thymus can be summarized as bringing about the differentiation and proliferation of primitive bone marrow-derived lymphoid cells and producing a humoral factor with the ability to induce immunological competence in lymphocytes. Immunologists are unfortunately as yet some way from understanding fully the exact mechanisms of interaction between the gland and the peripheral lymphoid tissues.

Gut-associated lymphoid tissue and antibody production

The thymus appears to control the cells of the cell-mediated immune system probably by providing facilities for the maturation of immature bone marrow cells. The cells of the immune system concerned with producing circulating antibodies reside mainly in the cortico-medullary junction and medullary cords of lymph nodes and the red pulp of the spleen. These cells, in contrast to those responsible for cell-mediated immunity, appear to be influenced not by the thymus but by lymphoid tissue associated with the intestine, namely in Peyer's patches and the appendix.

The first evidence that this might be so came from phylogenetic studies in neonatal chickens which failed to develop normal immunological capacity after removal of the gut-associated lymphoid organ known as the bursa of Fabricius. Thymectomized chickens, as would be expected from the discussion above, fail to develop cell-mediated immune processes whilst capable of a humoral immune response. In striking contrast, bursectomized chicken fail to make immunoglobulins and have no plasma cells or germinal centres in the lymphoid organs. Their cell-mediated mechanisms are, on the other hand, intact. Evidence is now emerging which suggests that there is a traffic of bursal lymphocytes to germinal centres in the spleen and lymph nodes comparable to that described in the thymus for bone marrow lymphocytes.

The search for an equivalent of the bursa in mammals, including man, is not yet complete but the evidence suggests that the lymphoid tissues of the appendix and Peyer's patches (and perhaps the tonsils) may perform this function.

Knowledge of immune-reactivity which is either thymus-dependent or bursa-dependent has led to the concept of separate *central* and *peripheral* lymphoid tissues. The central organs – the

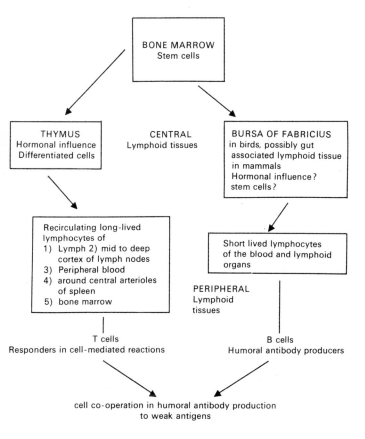

Fig. 17 Scheme illustrating possible relationship between central and peripheral lymphoid tissues.

thymus and the bursa of Fabricius (or its equivalent gut-associated tissue in mammals) – are responsible for development and control of the peripheral lymphoid tissues – the spleen and lymph nodes.

A tentative scheme showing the possible inter-relationships of central and peripheral lymphoid tissues is given in Figure 17. Recent work, based on repopulation of irradiated animals by lymphoid cells from different origins, indicates that for the expression of at least some forms of immune response, there may be co-operation between cells in the peripheral lymphoid tissues derived directly from the bone marrow and lymphocytes derived from the thymus. The former cells are referred to as B cells (bone marrow derived) and the latter as T cells (thymus-dependent). The B cells are believed to be responsible for immunoglobulin synthesis and may sometimes be directly stimulated by contact with antigen – usually powerful antigens such as salmonella flagellin or haemocyanin. Other weaker antigens such as serum albumin require the co-operation of T cells acting as helper cells leading in some way to an immune response by the B cells. Much more work is required before a clear picture emerges of the exact inter-relationship of these different cell populations.

Cellular Traffic in Other Lymphoid Tissues

In a previous section (p. 57) consideration was given to the traffic of lymphocytes from the bone marrow via the thymus to the lymph nodes. This journey, during which the cells are maturing and proliferating, probably takes a period of weeks. Another form of lymphocytic traffic also exists involving a population of short-lived (a few weeks) small lymphocytes, this journey being measured in hours rather than days (Fig. 18). This traffic takes the form of a recirculation of small lymphocytes between the blood and lymphoid tissue, and thus each small lymphocyte may be exchanged between these two compartments very many times during its lifetime. One of the main advantages to the individual of such a recirculation process is that, for example, during the course of a natural infection the continual traffic of lymphocytes would enable very many different lympho-cytes to have access to the antigen with the result that there

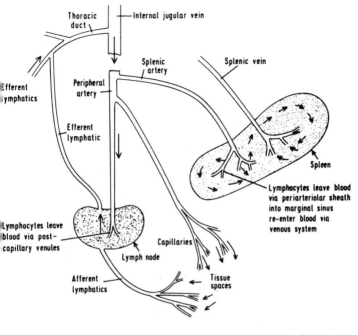

Fig. 18 Schematic view of main pathways of lymphocyte circulation.

would be a good chance that a lymphocyte carrying antibody receptor for the particular antigen would come across it and initiate an immune reaction. Another possible role of this re-circulation process is that it can be used to replenish the lymphoid tissue of, for example, the spleen which might have been depleted by X-irradiation, trauma or infection.

There is convincing evidence that lymphoid tissues can recruit lymphocytes from the recirculating pool. If a rat spleen is irradiated immediately after an intravenous injection of sheep red cells the antibody response is only slightly delayed. However if whole body irradiation is given after the initial splenic irradiation there is complete suppression of the anti-sheep cell response. It thus seems likely that without whole body irradiation the irradiated spleen is able to recruit a fresh supply of lymphocytes from the circulating pool.

Another situation in which recirculation of lymphocytes could be helpful in the induction of an immune response is where the local concentration of antigen might be sufficient to induce tolerance rather than immunity in a static cell population. The passage of lymphocytes through an area where antigen had been localized and concentrated on the dendritic processes of macrophages might facilitate the induction of immunity.

The routes of lymphocyte recirculation

There are three main areas where the migration or transfer of lymphocytes from the blood takes place: the lymph nodes and Peyer's patches, the spleen and the peripheral blood vessels. Most is known about the mechanism of transfer in the lymph nodes where studies using the electron microscope show that small lymphocytes actually penetrate and traverse the cytoplasm of the cuboidal endothelial cells of the post-capillary venules. These post-capillary venules are confined to the deep and mid zones of the lymph node cortex and are unusual in that their endothelial cells are hypertrophied and cuboidal in appearance in comparison with the flattened endothelium of normal post-capillary venules found elsewhere. From the lymph node cortex the lymphocytes pass through the node to the medullary sinuses and then to the efferent lymphatics.

The precise routes of lymphocyte migration in the peripheral blood circulation are not clear but the migration seems to be on a much smaller scale than in lymphoid tissues and almost certainly takes place across capillary walls. The flow can be increased if a local granuloma is formed in response to some foreign agent; then the migration from blood to lymph can be as great as in the lymph nodes themselves.

In the spleen, post-capillary venules have not been described and it appears that small lymphocytes enter the periarteriolar sheath from the blood, passing between the cells rather than through them as in the post-capillary venules. The cells later re-enter the blood within the spleen rather than leave via the lymphatics.

FURTHER READING

Barrett, J. T. (1970). *Textbook of Immunology*. London: Kimpton.

Burnet, Sir Macfarlane. (1969). *Cellular Immunity*. Cambridge University Press.

Cohen, S., Humphrey, J. H. & Coombs, R. R. A. (1967). Antibodies structure and biological function. *Proc. R. Soc. Med.* **60**, 589.

Cohen, S. & Milstein, C. (1967). Structure and biological properties of immunoglobulins. *Adv. Immun.* **7**, 1.

Dresser, D. W. & Mitchison, N. A. (1968). The mechanism of immunological paralysis. *Adv. Immun.* **8**, 129.

Edelman, G. M. (1970). The structure and function of antibodies. *Scient. Am.* **223**, 34.

Ford, W. L. & Gowans, J. L. (1969). The traffic of lymphocytes. *Semin. Hemat.* **6**, 67.

van Furth, R. (1970). *Mononuclear Phagocytes*. Oxford & Edinburgh: Blackwell.

Good, R. A., Finstad, J., Gewurz, H., Cooper, M. D. & Pollara, B. (1967). The development of immunological capacity in phylogenetic perspective. *Am. J. Dis. Child.* **114**, 477.

Hobbs, J. R. (1970). Immune globulins in some diseases. *Br. J. hosp. Med.* **3**, 669.

Holborow, E. J. (1968). *An ABC of Modern Immunology*. London: Lancet.

Humphrey, J. H. (1969). The fate of antigen and its relationship to the immune response. In *The Immune Response and its Suppression*. Ed. Sorkin, E. Basel: Karger.

Humphrey, J. H. & White, R. G. (1970). *Immunology for Students of Medicine*, 3rd ed. Oxford: Blackwell.

Kabat, E. A. (1968). *Structural Concepts in Immunology and Immunochemistry*. New York: Holt, Rinehart & Winston.

Mitchison, N. A. (1968). Immunological paralysis as a dosage phenomenon. In *Regulation of the Antibody Response*, p. 54. Ed. Cinader, B. Springfield, Illinois: Thomas.

Nossal, G. J. V. (1967). Mechanisms of antibody production. *A. Rev. Med.* **18**, 81.

Osaba, D. (1968). The regulatory role of the thymus in immunogenesis. In *Regulation of the Antibody Response*, p. 232. Ed. Cinader, B. Springfield, Illinois: Thomas.

Pinchuck, P. & Maurer, P. H. (1967). Genetic control of the immune response. In *Regulation of the Antibody Response*, p. 97. Ed. Cinader, B. Springfield, Illinois: Thomas.

Rogers Brambell, F. W. (1970). *The Transmission of Passive Immunity from Mother to Young*. Amsterdam: North Holland.

Smith, R. T. & Good, R. A. (1969). *Cellular Recognition*. New York: Appleton, Century & Crofts.

Smithies, O. (1968). Perspectives: mutation and selection in the immune system. In *Regulation of the Antibody Response*, p. 363. Ed. Cinader, B. Springfield, Illinois: Thomas.

Sorkin, E. (1968). *The Immune Response and its Suppression*. Basel: Karger.

Webb, T. &. Goodman, H. C. (1967). The structure and function of immuno-globulins. In *Modern Trends in Immunology*, 2, p. 151. Ed. Cruickshank, R. & Weir, D. M. London: Butterworth.

White, R. G. (1967). Antigen adjuvants. In *Modern Trends in Immunology*, 2, p. 28. Ed. Cruickshank, R. & Weir, D. M. London: Butterworth.

Wigzell, H. (1967). Studies in the regulation of antibody synthesis. *Cold Spring Harbor Symp. quant. Biol.* **32,** 507.

Wolstenholme, G. E. W. & Knight, J. (1970). *Hormones and the Immune Response*. Ciba Foundation Study Group No. 36. London: Churchill.

Chapter 5

DEFECTS IN IMMUNOGLOBULIN SYNTHESIS AND CELL-MEDIATED IMMUNE REACTIVITY

The immunologically competent cells of the lymphoid tissues derived from, renewed and influenced by the activity of the thymus, bone marrow and probably gut-associated lymphoid tissues, can be the subject of disease processes due either to defects in one of the components of the complex itself or secondarily to some other disease process affecting the normal functioning of some part of the lymphoid tissues. In 1953 Bruton first described hypogammaglobulinaemia in an 8-year-old boy who developed septic arthritis of the knee at 4 years of age followed by numerous attacks of otitis media, pneumococcal sepsis and pneumonia. Electrophoretic analysis of the serum proteins showed almost complete absence of the gamma-globulin fraction. The child appeared unable to give an immune response to typhoid and diphtheria immunization. It is now recognized that this form of deficiency is only one of a group of specific deficiencies affecting the lymphoid tissues which can affect both sexes, manifest themselves at any age and be genetically determined or arise secondarily to some other condition.

Primary defects

In the first category are the congenital defects affecting immunoglobulin synthetic mechanisms, cell-mediated immune mechanisms or sometimes both. Deficiency of immunoglobulin synthesis is complete in Bruton type agammaglobulinaemia an X-linked recessive character found in boys and in which the IgG level is reduced about tenfold and the IgA and IgM about a hundredfold normal values. Cell-mediated immune mechanisms function normally in these patients who can reject grafts and develop normal delayed hypersensitivity to tuberculosis. However they do not give the normal circulating antibody response to bacterial vaccines and are thus very susceptible to pyogenic infections. The lymphoid tissue in the appendix and Peyer's patches is somewhat reduced, and patients do not develop plasma cells and germinal centres in lymph nodes.

Partial defects in immunoglobulin synthesis have been described affecting one or more of the main immunoglobulin classes. For example (a) the IgG or IgA levels may be reduced and the IgM level raised; (b) the IgA and IgM may be reduced and the IgG level be normal or (c) the IgA level may be reduced and the others normal.

In (a), which is also inherited as an X-linked recessive character, the lymphoid tissues appear normal histologically although the plasma cells appear to be making predominantly IgM. Patients are susceptible to pyogenic infections and the condition is often associated with anaemia, thrombocytopoenia and neutropoenia. In (b) even the IgG which is produced in normal quantity is thought to be abnormal in some way and unable to combine with antigen. Defect (c) occurs in 80 per cent of patients with a condition known as hereditary ataxia telangiectasia who have increased susceptibility to infections of the upper and lower respiratory tract. There is a deficiency in plasma cells in the mucous membranes of the intestinal tract, where IgA is known to be produced in normal individuals, and the disease seems likely to be due to lack of protection at the level of the respiratory mucous membranes normally brought about by IgA secretion.

Both *cell-mediated* immune mechanisms and *immunoglobulin synthesis* are deficient in an X-linked disease of male children known as 'Swiss type agammaglobulinaemia'. There is almost complete absence of lymphoid tissue in the body, the thymus is very small and the lymphoid tissues of the appendix and Peyer's patches are absent. Children with this condition cannot make antibodies or develop cell-mediated immune reactions, and they suffer from progressive bacterial and/or viral infection and die within two years of birth.

In another type of deficiency state only the cell-mediated immune mechanisms are affected and there is thymic dysplasia and deficiency of lymphoid cells from those areas of the spleen and lymph nodes which are under thymic control. Although children with this rare type of deficiency can produce circulating antibody their inability to develop cell-mediated immunity renders them highly susceptible to virus infection. One form of this condition associated with thymic dysplasia and absence of parathyroid glands is known as Di George's syndrome.

Secondary defects

Acquired deficiencies of the immunological mechanisms can occur secondarily to a number of disease states affecting the lymphoid tissues such as Hodgkin's disease, multiple myeloma, leukaemia and lymphosarcoma. Deficiency of immunoglobulins can also be brought about by excessive loss of protein through diseased kidneys or via the intestines in protein-losing enteropathy. In contrast to the deficiency state just described, raised immunoglobulin levels are found in certain disorders of plasma cell function, which amount to malignant proliferation of a particular clone or family of plasma cells. In this condition known as multiple myeloma, a malignant clone is found to produce one particular class of immunoglobulin usually IgG or more rarely one of the other classes. The frequency of occurrence among myeloma of particular immunoglobulin classes reflects their relative levels in serum. There is usually a decreased synthesis of normal immunoglobulins associated with a deficient immune response to infective agents. On electrophoresis of serum a distinct band can be seen in the immunoglobulin area. This abnormal band is produced by the raised levels of the myeloma immunoglobulin which is termed an M-type protein. In about 20–30 per cent of patients with multiple myeloma immunoglobulin light chains are found in the urine. These occur as dimers and are known as Bence-Jones protein. The condition is also associated with excess numbers of plasma cells in the bone marrow and X-ray evidence of myeloma cell deposits in bone.

Clinical aspects

Increased susceptibility to many types of infection is the outstanding feature of the immunological deficiency states. The age of onset of the congenital types is rarely earlier than 3–4 months of age due to the protective effects of maternal antibody. The most frequently affected site is the respiratory tract which is attacked by pyogenic bacteria or fungi. Lack of IgA antibody leads to particular susceptibility to chronic infection of the respiratory tract.

When there is deficiency of the cell-mediated immune mechanisms resistance to virus infections is diminished which may be recognized by the severe necrosis that will occur at the site of smallpox vaccination. BCG vaccination can lead to generalized tuberculosis infection in such cases.

Investigation of suspected immunological deficiency states should include family studies for any abnormalities of immune function, quantitative determination of immunoglobulin levels and estimation of the response to immunization with standard antigens. Peripheral blood counts and X-rays of the thymus region may also prove useful.

Treatment of deficiency states includes use of an appropriate antibiotic and regular administration of pooled human immunoglobulins. Closely matched sibling bone marrow has been used successfully in some cases and a graft of foetal thymus has been used in the case of thymic aplasia.

Defective Phagocytic Mechanisms

These defects take two forms. (1) Where there is a *quantitative* deficiency of blood leucocytes which may be *congenital* (e.g. infantile agranulocytosis) or *acquired* as a result of replacement of bone marrow by tumour tissue or the toxic effects of chemicals. (2) Where there is a *qualitative* deficiency in the functioning of neutrophil leucocytes which whilst ingesting bacteria normally fail, because of an enzymic defect, to digest them. The clinical form of this defect is known as chronic granulomatous disease and is a sex-linked recessive condition characterized by increased susceptibility to infection in early life by microorganisms of low virulence to the normal individual.

FURTHER READING

Martin, N. H. (1970). The paraproteinaemias. *Br. J. hosp. Med.,* **3,** 662.

Soothill, J. F. (1968). Immunity deficiency states. In *Clinical Aspects of Immunology,* 2nd ed. Ed. Gell, P. G. H. & Coombs, R. R. A. Oxford: Blackwell.

Turk, J. L. (1969). *Immunology in Clinical Medicine.* London: Heinemann.

Waldenstrom, J. G. (1968). *Monoclonal and Polyclonal Hypergammaglobulinemia – Clinical and Biological Significance.* Cambridge University Press.

Chapter 6

HYPERSENSITIVITY

Since immunity was first recognized as a resistant state that
followed infection, immunology developed primarily as an aspect
of medical bacteriology with emphasis on acquired specific
resistance to invasion by microorganisms as a means of
protection against infection. Much of the present terminology
originates from this early period in the development of
immunology. The term immunity, meaning safe or exempt, has
now been extended far beyond its early meaning and includes
reactions to foreign material such as grafted tissues, blood
products and various bland chemical substances none of which
bears any relation to infectious agents. Some forms of immune
reaction rather than providing exemption or safety to the
affected individual can produce severe and occasionally fatal
results. These are known as 'hypersensitivity reactions' and in
the main are due to tissue damage caused by effects of pharmacologically active agents such as histamine which are formed
under certain conditions of antigen-antibody combination.

The term allergy was originally coined by von Pirquet early
this century to describe the altered reactivity of an animal
following exposure to a foreign antigen, and included both
immunity and hypersensitivity. The term, however, has over the
years become restricted to refer only to the hypersensitivity
which may be associated with the development of the immune
response to a foreign substance.

Immediate and delayed hypersensitivity

There are two main forms of hypersensitivity reaction:
immediate and *delayed* (Fig. 19). The immediate form appears
rapidly and depends on the production of pharmacologically
active mediator substances activated by antigen-antibody interaction. The delayed form appears more slowly (usually after 24

hours) and depends on immunologically activated lymphoid cells which on reaction with antigen appear to release substances known as lymphokines having a variety of effects on other cells and effects on blood vessel permeability (p. 78).

Various classifications of hypersensitivity reactions have been

Exposure to foreign antigenic material

(infective or bland) — — — — — — — — — — — — — — — ► Protective against infective agent

HYPERSENSITIVITY

Disadvantageous reaction

Immediate type, antibody-mediated (types 1–3)

Delayed type, cell-mediated (type 4)

Fig. 19 Hypersensitivity reactions

proposed and probably the most widely accepted is that of Coombs and Gell. This recognizes four types or categories of hypersensitivity reactions, three of which come under the heading of immediate reactions: type 1, anaphylactic reactions; type 2, cytolytic or cytotoxic reactions; and type 3, toxic-complex syndrome. The fourth type is the cell-mediated delayed hypersensitivity form of reaction.

Anaphylactic reactions of type 1

If a guinea-pig is injected with a small dose of an antigen such as egg albumen no adverse effects are noted. If however, a second injection of the egg albumen antigen is given intravenously after an interval of about 10 days a condition known as 'anaphylactic shock' is likely to develop. The animal becomes restless, starts chewing and rubbing its nose with its front paws, respiration becomes laboured, the animal becomes cyanosed and may develop convulsions and die. The initial injection of antigen is termed the 'sensitizing dose' and the second injection the 'shocking dose'. During the interval between the two injections the animal has formed antibody and anaphylaxis is the result of interaction of the shocking dose of antigen with antibody which triggers the release of pharmacologically active substances causing increase in capillary permeability and contraction of smooth muscle in many parts of the body. In the guinea-pig this particularly affects the smooth muscles of the bronchioles causing respiratory embarrassment.

Pharmacological mediators

Four pharmacologically active substances have been implicated to varying degrees in anaphylactic reactions: (1) histamine, (2) 5-hydroxy-tryptamine, (3) slow-reacting substance, (4) the bradykinins. Predominant amongst these and responsible for many of the symptoms of anaphylactic shock is *histamine* which can be shown to be liberated *in vitro* when antibody-sensitized pieces of various tissues including uterine muscle, lung and intestine are exposed to contact with antigen. Sensitization may be produced by prior injection of antigen into the animal supplying the tissue which makes antibody as described above or the tissue may be sensitized passively by the addition of antibody produced in another animal. The typical contractions induced in this way in the uterus and intestine are called Schultze-Dale reactions after the originators. The histamine is derived from the granules of mast cells where it exists as its precursor histidine, in combination with heparin; these substances are released by the interaction of antigen with antibody via another pharmacologically active substance anaphylatoxin acting together with serum complement components (p. 13).

The eosinophil is thought to play an important part in anaphylactic reactions, many of these marrow-derived cells being found in the blood and tissues during an anaphylactic reaction. Exactly what role these cells play is uncertain but one suggestion is that they are attracted by released histamine and take part in its detoxification.

The other pharmacological mediators of immediate hypersensitivity reactions are: 5-hydroxy-tryptamine or serotonin which causes contraction of plain muscle and increased capillary permeability. It is of uncertain role in anaphylaxis, although it is probably involved in local intestinal food allergies; slow-reacting substance (or SRS-A) has a plain muscle contracting effect acting, unlike histamine, on the larger rather than smaller blood vessels. SRS-A has a particularly marked bronchial constricting effect in man and is probably the predominant pharmacological agent in human asthma. Bradykinins are simple peptides formed from a plasma α globulin (kininogen) by plasma kinin-forming enzymes. They have histamine-like effects on smooth muscle and capillaries, and studies have shown that it is present in the blood stream in many species in the early stages of an anaphylactic reaction.

Systemic and local forms

In man there are two types of anaphylactic reaction – *systemic* and *local* – and which one of these develops depends on how the shocking dose of antigen enters the body. The systemic form of anaphylaxis is likely to develop if antigen is injected parenterally, as in the case of foreign serum (e.g. horse anti-tetanus serum), or a drug such as penicillin, or perhaps by the bite of an insect. The symptoms include dyspnoea with bronchospasm and laryngeal oedema, sometimes skin rashes, a fall in blood pressure and occasionally death. If on the other hand, the antigen comes in contact with respiratory mucous membranes, then in a sensitized individual the local forms of anaphylaxis will develop - i.e. hay fever or asthma. If the intestinal mucous membrane of a susceptible individual comes in contact with the appropriate antigen (e.g. nuts, fish or strawberries), then a mixed form of reaction can develop with intestinal symptoms, skin rashes (urticaria) and sometimes the symptoms of asthma.

The antibodies involved in anaphylactic reactions

The role of IgE

In the human the antibodies which sensitize the tissues for anaphylactic reactions have been known for many years as *reaginic* antibodies. These antibodies have a strong affinity for tissues and can readily be detected in the serum of a sensitized individual by injecting a small quantity of the serum into the skin of a normal recipient, and 24–48 hours later, introducing the appropriate antigen into the injection site. Within about 20 minutes a weal and flare erythematous reaction develops at the injection site, just like the response to an injection of histamine. This reaction is called the P.K. test after its originators Prausnitz and Küstner.

The nature of reaginic antibody was not finally elucidated until late in 1967 when a hitherto undescribed form of myeloma protein was discovered in Sweden although work in America suggested the existence of an immunoglobulin distinct from IgG, IgM or IgA. This made it possible (using an antiserum prepared in a sheep to the myeloma globulin) to show in normal human serum a new class of immunoglobulin present in very low concentration (0.0001–0.0007 mg/100 ml of serum cf. 900–1800 mg of IgG/100 ml serum). The skin sensitizing activity of reaginic antibody could readily be neutralized by means of the antiserum to this new immunoglobulin which has been named IgE (for discussion of its structure see p. 47). The concentration of IgE in patients with allergic asthma has been found to be much higher than in normal individuals. The comparatively low levels of IgE found in serum presumably reflect the affinity of this immunoglobulin for tissues so that freshly made IgE is very soon removed from serum when it comes in contact with the appropriate cell receptors on mast cells and possibly elsewhere.

Immunological approaches to the prevention of anaphylaxis

Blocking antibody

On consideration of the mechanism of systemic anaphylaxis it would seem likely that if the parenterally injected antigen could be prevented from reaching the tissue-fixed IgE then anaphylaxis would not develop. This desirable state of affairs can be achieved by the simple expedient of injecting frequent small doses of the antigen to which the patient is sensitized. This induces the formation of increasing levels of IgG antibody which, circulating in the blood and tissue fluids, mops up the injected antigen so that it does not reach the tissue-fixed IgE (Fig. 20). This IgG antibody has been termed *blocking antibody* and its

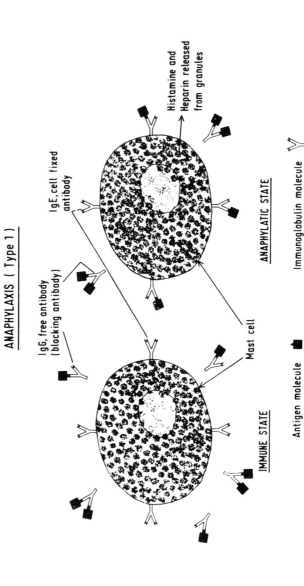

ANAPHYLAXIS (Type 1)

IgG, free antibody (blocking antibody)

IgE. cell fixed antibody

Histamine and Heparin released from granules

Mast cell

IMMUNE STATE

ANAPHYLATIC STATE

Antigen molecule ▪   Immunoglobulin molecule ⅄

Fig. 20 Diagrammatic view of the possible difference between an 'immune state' (i.e. when immunized animal will not develop anaphylaxis on challenge with antigen) and an 'anaphylactic state'. Here there is insufficient antibody free in the tissue fluids to mop up the antigen thus allowing it to combine with reaginic antibody (IgE) attached to cell. The interaction triggers the release of histamine and heparin from mast cell granules.

induction is the basis of desensitization treatment in allergic individuals. As might be expected this method is much more effective in preventing systemic anaphylactic reactions than the local forms where the antigen does not enter the blood stream. To prevent local anaphylaxis the blocking antibody would need to be present in the mucous secretions and parenteral injection of antigen is hardly the best way to achieve this (see p. 96 for discussion of immunization against influenza virus).

In theory it should be possible by raising the level of IgE to antigens other than those responsible for the allergic sensitization to occupy the tissue receptors by non-specific IgE antibodies rather than those formed to the sensitizing antigen. Whether such a procedure is feasible remains to be established.

Cytolytic or cytotoxic (type 2) reactions

Cell-associated antigens

Reactions of this type are initiated by an antigenic component either part of a tissue cell or closely associated with it (e.g. a drug attached to the cell wall (Fig. 21)). The antibodies directed against such a cell-associated antigen bring about a cytotoxic or cytolytic effect usually involving complement. Reactions of this type include the cytolytic effect of anti-red cell antibodies, induced by incompatible blood transfusion, on the foreign erythrocytes. Haemolytic disease of the newborn has a similar mechanism as do certain forms of auto-immune haemolytic anaemia in which the patient forms antibodies against auto-logous red cells. There are many examples of these cytotoxic or cytolytic reactions which are brought about by an immune reaction to a foreign substance which becomes attached to the cell membranes of erythrocytes, leucocytes or platelets. One of the best known examples of this phenomenon is Sedormid purpura (apronal). The complexing of the drug Sedormid with platelets results in an antibody response directed against the platelet-adsorbed drug which brings about destruction of the platelets and purpura. As a result of the elucidation of the mechanism of this disease by Ackroyd in London, Sedormid has been withdrawn from use. This type of reaction may be more widespread than is generally suspected. A variety of infectious diseases due to salmonella organisms and mycobacteria are

Foreign Red cells

Drug or substance derived from infectious agent coats patients red cells

Stimulates antibody response

in presence of complement

Agglutination, lysis and cell destruction

Fig. 21 Cytolytic and cytotoxic (type 2) reactions

associated with haemolytic anaemia, and there is evidence, particularly in studies in salmonella infections, that the haemolysis is due to an immune reaction against a lipopolysaccharide bacterial endotoxin which becomes coated on to the patient's erythrocytes. A detailed study of *Salmonella gallinarum* infection in chickens has shown conclusively that the red cells are coated, have a shorter life in the circulation due to haemolysis and that the development of haemolysis directly parallels the level of the anti-lipopolysaccharide antibody.

Toxic-complex syndrome (type 3) reactions

Serum sickness and Arthus reactions

These reactions are due to the combination of antigen with circulating antibody with the formation of microprecipitates in and around small blood vessels causing inflammation and some-times mechanical blocking of these vessels which results in interference with the blood supply to surrounding tissues. There are two types of reaction which fall into this category: *serum sickness* which is a systemic form and the *Arthus reaction* which is a local form. Serum sickness develops, as the name suggests, in individuals injected with foreign serum and was described soon after the introduction of parenteral administration for thera-peutic purposes of diphtheria antitoxin prepared in the horse. Foreign serum protein is eliminated from the circulation over a period of a few weeks and after the injection of 10–20 ml there will still be a large amount present by the time an immune response to the foreign serum protein develops. This results in the formation of antibody-antigen complexes that can cause a wide variety of symptoms ranging from anaphylactic reactions such as asthma or laryngeal oedema when IgE antibody attached to mast cells is involved, to symptoms dependent on the de-position of immune complexes (antigen + IgG antibody) in blood vessels where they activate complement and cause inflammatory changes. The organs affected are the kidney, with the development of glomerulonephritis and in severe cases renal failure, the heart, with myocarditis and valvulitis, and the joints which become swollen and painful. Urticaria sometimes develops and the patient becomes pyrexial. The symptoms disappear whenever all the foreign serum protein is eliminated. Antigens other than serum proteins can cause serum sickness. Nowadays the most likely causes are drugs such as penicillin and sulpho-namides.

The Arthus reaction like serum sickness is brought about by the formation of antibody-antigen complexes but in this case the phenomenon is a local one at the site of injection of antigen. The Arthus reaction occurs in walls of small blood vessels in the presence of large quantities of IgG antibody forming micro-precipitates with antigen. The resulting vasculitis develops a few hours after injection of antigen and persists for 12–24 hours.

Immune complexes can be shown microscopically in the vessel wall using the fluorescent antibody technique (p. 144) and there is a massive infiltration of granulocytes brought about by a chemotactic effect generated by the antigen-antibody complex. There is activation of the vasoactive amines such as histamine, with resulting increase in vascular permeability and consequent oedema. These reactions are of relatively minor clinical importance but may occur in diabetics who have received many injections of insulin and have developed high levels of IgG antibody to antigenic constituents in the insulin preparation.

Delayed Hypersensitivity, (type 4) cell-mediated hypersensitivity

Lymphocyte-mediated reactions and 'lymphokines'

These can be defined as specifically provoked, slowly evolving (24–48 hours) mixed cellular reactions involving particularly lymphocytes and macrophages. The reaction is not brought about by circulating antibody but by sensitized lymphoid cells and can be transferred in experimental animals by means of such cells but not by serum. The classical example of this type of reaction is the tuberculin response which has over the years received detailed study. To induce this response a tuberculin-sensitized individual is given an intradermal injection of 0.1 ml of a 1 in 1000 dilution of a protein extract of tubercle bacilli (purified protein derivative PPD). An indurated inflammatory reaction in the skin, measuring a few millimetres in diameter, appears about 24 hours later and persists for a few weeks. In the human the injection site is infiltrated with large numbers of mononuclear cells, mainly lymphocytes, with about 10–20 per cent macrophages. Most of these cells are in or around small blood vessels. Despite intensive investigation of the delayed hypersensitivity reaction immunologists are far from understanding the mechanisms underlying this phenomenon. A possible explanation is that amongst the continuous traffic of lymphocytes passing through the tissues (p. 61) there are some sensitized cells possibly with 'antibody-like receptors' on their surface. These cells interact with antigen they meet and in some unknown way influence other lymphocytes to migrate to the area.

In the last few years a group of as yet ill-defined substances have been shown to be released by lymphocytes coming in contact with the antigen to which they have been sensitized. The name *lymphokines* has been proposed to describe this group of non-antibody lymphocyte factors. The chemotactic factor mentioned above attracting additional lymphocytes to the site of localization of antigen is one of the lymphokines. Another factor appears to be responsible for inducing proliferation of lymphocytes at the site of localization and has been termed mitogenic factor. A cytotoxic effect has been demonstrated in tissue culture experiments affecting lymphocytes and other cells (lymphotoxin). The best known of the lymphokines is the macrophage migration inhibition factor. This effect is readily demonstrated *in vitro* using peritoneal exudate cells from an animal sensitized to an antigen such as tuberculin. The peritoneal exudate cells which are mainly macrophages are collected in a capillary tube that is placed on a glass coverslip in a small tissue culture chamber (Fig. 8). After 24 hours macrophages show a fan-shaped area of migration around the end of the capillary tube. If however, the tuberculin antigen is placed in the tissue culture medium no migration occurs. The effect appears to be due to the release from the small number of lymphocytes in peritoneal exudate of a lymphokine known as macrophage migration inhibition factor or MIF. The specificity of the reaction has been shown with several other antigens including bovine gamma globulin, histoplasmin and dinitrophenol. The MIF appears to be released from cells concerned with the cell-mediated immune state rather than cells concerned with making humoral antibody. The chemical nature of MIF has not yet been established although it appears in guinea pigs to have an MW of about 70,000 (like some of the other lymphokines) and is susceptible to proteolytic enzymes. *In vivo* the factor may be responsible for the formation of large aggregates of macrophages in the lymphoid tissues (and perhaps elsewhere), although like the other lymphokines the precise role of MIF in delayed hypersensitivity reaction is not yet clear and much further work is required to separate and identify the nature and functional activities of the various substances involved. Whether or not macrophages in delayed hypersensitivity reaction sites contribute lysosomal enzymes from their intracellular granules thus bringing about further inflammatory changes has yet to be determined.

Inducing agents

Delayed hypersensitivity reactions are characteristically induced by intracellular infectious agents including salmonellae, brucellae, streptococci and a wide range of viruses including measles and mumps viruses, vaccinia and herpes simplex. Those with most clinical relevance are reactions due to vaccinia – the so-called 'reaction of immunity' occurring 24–72 hours after vaccination. This reaction does not proceed like a primary vaccination through the pustular stage and leaves no scar but instead has all the features of a delayed hypersensitivity reaction. The other important reaction is the 'pseudo-Schick' response occurring within 24 hours after the intradermal injection of diphtheria toxoid. This delayed response disappears within six days and also affects the control injected site (heat-treated toxoid). Delayed hypersensitivity reactions sometimes develop following sensitization to a variety of metals such as nickel and chromium, to simple chemical substances such as dyestuffs, potassium dichromate (affecting cement workers), primulin from primula plants, poison ivy and chemicals such as picryl chloride, dinitrochloro-benzene, and paraphenylene diamine (from hair dyes). Penicillin sensitization is a common clinical complication following the topical application of the antibiotic in ointments or creams. These substances are not themselves antigenic and only become so on combination by covalent bonds with proteins in the skin. The clinical symptoms induced in these 'contact hypersensitivity' reactions (contact dermatitis) include redness, swelling, vesicles, scaling and exudation of fluid.

It is conceivable that in the future, use may be made of the delayed hypersensitivity response in the treatment of tumours. Some recent experiments in man show that certain skin tumours, if painted with a simple chemical antigen as described above, underwent a marked hypersensitivity reaction and then healed with the disappearance of the tumour. One explanation of the effect is that the lymphokine—lymphotoxin—is released during the hypersensitivity reaction and destroys the tumour cells. Much more work is clearly required before this can be regarded as a useful clinical procedure.

FURTHER READING

Austen, F. J. & Block, K. J. (1968). *Biochemistry of Acute Allergic Reactions.* Oxford: Blackwell.

Gell, P. G. H. & Coombs, R. R. A. (1968). The allergic state as responsible for clinical hypersensitivity and disease. In *Clinical Aspects of Immunology,* 2nd ed., Sect. IV. Oxford: Blackwell.

Turk, J. L. (1967). Delayed hypersensitivity. In *Frontiers in Biology,* Vol. 4. Ed. Neuberger, A. & Tatum, E. L. Amsterdam: North Holland.

Turk, J. L. (1967). Delayed hypersensitivity – specific cell-mediated immunity. *Br. med. Bull.* **23,** No. 1.

Turk, J. L. (1969). *Immunology in Clinical Medicine.* London: Heinemann.

Uhr, J. W. (1966). Delayed hypersensitivity. *Physiol. Rev.,* **46,** 359.

Chapter 7

THE IMMUNOLOGY OF TISSUE TRANSPLANTATION

The tissue cells of animals contain antigens that are specific for the species of origin of the cell, and which if implanted into an animal of another species will induce an immune response. This response rapidly destroys the implanted cells and has the characteristics of the primary and secondary immune response as already described for antigens in general. In addition to species

Table 4 Transplantation terminology
(older terminology in brackets)

Relationship between donor and recipient	Term applied to relationship	Prefix applied to graft, antigen or antibody
Of different species	Xenogeneic (heterogeneic)	Xeno- (hetero-)
Of same species but different genetic constitution	Allogeneic (homologous)	Allo- (homo-)
Of same inbred strain	Syngeneic (isogeneic) (isologous)	—
Same individual	Autologous	Auto-

specific antigens, differences also exist between individual members of the same species so that transfer of tissue cells between members induces a similar immune reaction. The closer the relationship between two individuals of the same species the more likely are implanted cells to survive and in the case of identical twins survival is assured. Inbred strains of animals, particularly mice, have been developed which are genetically identical and these are widely used in experimental work on tissue transplantation immunology.

In man surgical techniques are available to enable transplantation of many organs and tissues but unfortunately a high proportion of organ transplants fail because of rejection by the immune response or because of the side effects of attempts to suppress the immune response, due to toxicity of the drugs or their depressive effect on resistance to infection.

Transplantation antigen systems

The first systematic studies on the antigens carried by cells which determine whether a graft will be rejected or not were carried out in inbred strains of mice of known genetic make up.

It was found that there were very many antigenic differences between tissues of different strains of mice, the number of separate antigens involved being estimated at between 15 and 500 in different experiments. However it was found that, just as in the red cell antigenic system, some antigens were very 'strong' and others very weak. The strong transplantation or 'histocompatibility' antigens of the mouse are controlled by the H-2 genetic locus and in man by the HL-A locus.

The mouse H-2 system appears to consist of a system of closely linked genes and there are hundreds of possible combinations resulting in different H-2 antigens. H-2 antigens are found in large amounts in epithelium and lymphoid tissues, in very small amounts in kidney or muscle and are virtually absent from brain and testis.

In man, two strong and several weak histocompatibility systems have been found. As mentioned already the HL-A is the strong system with the ABH blood group system next in importance. The major loci are very complex, the antigens being determined by a chromosomal region rather than by a single genetic locus.

Leucocyte grouping

The strong antigens of the HL-A system are widely distributed in the tissues but absent from the red blood cells which contain only the ABH antigens.

Fortunately blood leucocytes carry all the known HL-A

antigens and it is therefore possible to test for the presence or absence of antigens of the system using leucocyte agglutination and cytotoxicity tests (p. 147). In principle the leuco-agglutination test is performed with leucocytes separated from the erythrocytes of anticoagulant-treated blood. Specific antisera for HL-A antigens are then used to agglutinate the leucocytes and the tests are read under the microscope. The cytotoxic test is carried out with a purified suspension of blood lymphocytes which are mixed with antisera to HL-A antigens in the presence of complement (p. 12). If the lymphocytes carry the appropriate antigens the antiserum will combine and in the presence of complement will damage the cell membrane. The resulting increased cell membrane permeability is usually detected by dye uptake into the cell.

Despite the very great diversity among HL-A alleles of unrelated subjects it is encouraging to find that about a third of kidneys from unrelated donors survive for a year or longer although only a third of them show normal kidney function. Although this partial success must be dependent to an extent on the use of immunosuppressive agents differences in the 'strength' of individual HL-A antigens is probably partly responsible.

Mechanisms of graft rejection

There are two main types of graft rejection process: (a) the so-called 'first set' response which occurs about 10 days after a first graft from an unrelated donor, (b) the 'second set' response occurring in about 7 days in an animal which had previously received a graft from the same unrelated donor. This phenomenon of first and second set rejection can be compared to primary and secondary immunization – the accelerated secondary response being brought about by stimulation of an already sensitized or 'primed' immune system.

The role of lymphoid cells

It can be shown histologically that grafts undergoing rejection are heavily infiltrated with lymphocytes and that there is extensive vascular damage. Other types of cell of the immune system, such as plasma cells and macrophages, are also frequently found in association with graft rejection. The ability to reject grafts can readily be transferred from one animal to another by a process known as *adoptive transfer* of lymphoid cells from an immune animal (i.e. one capable of a second set graft rejection) to a non-immune recipient of the same strain. Lymphoid cells appear to be able to transfer this ability most effectively when taken before the circulating antibody level reaches its peak. Contrary to expectation, it is possible to show, using isotope-labelled cells, that it is not the transferred cells which migrate to the graft but those of the recipient, the donated cells in the main homing to the lymphoid organs, as no more are found in the graft than at control sites. It is however possible that those few donated cells which settle in the graft area are cells specifically sensitized to the graft antigens whilst those settling out elsewhere are the unsensitized cells. From what is known about the recirculating lymphocyte pool (p. 61) it seems likely that there is a good chance of cells with a specific ability to react to an antigen coming in contact with such material in a graft during the recirculation process.

The role of circulating antibody

The ability to reject grafts cannot be transferred from one animal to another by means of passively injected antibody. This does not rule out the possibility that antibody can play a part in graft rejection, because when the serum, containing at best about 1 per cent specific antibody, is injected into a recipient the diluting effect of the blood and tissue fluids considerably reduces the possibility of the antibody reaching the graft site in an adequate concentration to influence the viability of the graft. The same antibody-containing serum can readily be shown *in vitro* to be cytotoxic, in the presence of complement, for cells containing antigens to which the antibody was produced. However this is an artificial situation and does not take into account the dilution effects discussed above. Kidney grafts which have survived for some time, perhaps months or years, can, it seems, be rejected by serum antibody alone without any evidence of invasion of the graft by lymphoid cells. Deposits of immunoglobulin and complement can be detected particularly in the walls of blood vessels. Although at this stage no antibodies may be detected in the serum, if the rejected kidney is removed they soon appear, suggesting that the antibodies were rapidly removed by combination with kidney antigens. The kidney is rejected by the development of a progressive vasculitis affecting glomerular and other vessels.

Locally produced antibody and non-antibody lymphocyte factors

The possibility is quite strong that antibody made locally in a graft by the infiltrating lymphoid cells is present in a sufficiently high concentration in the area immediately surrounding the antibody-producing cell to damage incompatible cells of the graft. This situation can be compared to the observation made *in vitro* with the Jerne plaque technique (p. 26) in which lymphocytes can be shown to be producing antibody to sheep red blood cells which produces a surrounding halo of lysis of the red cells in the presence of complement. Indeed, lymphocytes and plasma cells invading grafts can be shown to contain immunoglobulin. Evidence that immunoglobulin is combining with antigen during graft rejection is provided by a detectable fall in the serum complement level. There are a number of other possible direct ways in which the infiltrating lymphocytes can influence survival of the graft: (a) the antibody which they produce may activate the various pharmacological mediators of immediate hypersensitivity reactions such as histamine (p. 71) and these will bring about vascular changes in the vessels of the graft; (b) the lymphocytes on contact with antigen may release macrophage migration inhibition factor (MIF) (p. 33) which will cause accumulation of macrophages in the graft; (c) it is known that sensitized lymphocytes can influence non-immune lymphocytes to behave aggressively towards cells in their vicinity and induce cytotoxic effects. How this is brought about is not clear but may conceivably depend upon the release of one of the factors mentioned above.

It can thus be seen that the reaction against a graft depends upon a complex series of interrelated phenomena some of which are specifically induced by the foreign nature of graft antigens. Other phenomena are non-specific in the immunological sense and occur as part of an inflammatory process.

Immunosuppression

Graft rejection, as has been noted, involves a sequence of

86

separate phenomena developing from initial contact of the foreign antigens with the host immunological system through to rejection itself. The steps include establishment of lymphatic drainage, antigen release, its contact with cells of the immune system, proliferation of antibody-forming cells of the lymphoid tissues, the inflammatory response and release of pharmacological mediators and cytotoxic effects of lymphoid cells and/or antibody on the graft tissues.

Prevention of sensitization; tolerance to graft antigens

Interference with any of these stages would be likely to interfere with the rejection process. One of the most interesting approaches, which is as yet unfortunately only at the experimental stage, is interference with what might be termed the afferent arc of the process of rejection, namely the initial sensitization of the lymphoid cells. If it were possible to induce immune tolerance (p. 50) to the strong histocompatibility antigens of tissue grafts, then clearly immunological rejection would not take place. The tolerant animal although unable to react against the antigen to which it is tolerant can still respond to other antigens such as potentially infective agents like bacteria, fungi or viruses; this obviates one of the greatest difficulties associated with immunosuppressive procedures (p. 88).

As has been noted earlier, Mitchison (using serum protein antigens) has shown that there are two types of tolerance, so-called 'high dose' tolerance where the immune system is overloaded with excess antigen, and 'low dose' tolerance where only minute quantities of antigen are administered. Although the molecular processes underlying these phenomena are not as yet understood, clearly the 'low dose' tolerance phenomenon has great potential application to transplantation problems. When it becomes possible to extract purified transplantation antigens from tissue, it should then be possible to prepare an individual for graft acceptance by inducing low dose tolerance to the appropriate antigens.

Immunological enhancement

Another phenomenon relevant to the maintenance of incompatible grafts is 'immunological enhancement'. This is brought about by antibody produced against graft antigens that can under certain circumstances protect the graft from attack by cells of the immune system. This system has been used successfully in rats with incompatible kidney grafts, the animals being previously immunized with tissue from the prospective donor. The grafts exhibit normal renal function for a year or more afterwards. The method has been applied in a few instances to human kidney grafts and the results suggest that the method may be of considerable future value. The mechanism may involve coating of the cells of the graft by non-complement-fixing antibody and/or direct inhibition of antibody production against the graft brought about by the antibody.

Practical approaches

In practice there are at the moment three main approaches to the problem of immunosuppression: (1) X-irradation to knock out the lymphoid tissues and abolish the immune response; (2) immuno-suppressive drugs – antimetabolites and anti-inflammatory agents to prevent proliferation of antibody-forming cells; (3) immunological methods – anti-lymphocyte serum (ALS) produced, for example, in the horse, to attack the lymphocytes directly and destroy them before they attack the graft.

Whole body X-irradiation used in the early days of organ transplantation has been replaced in the main by immuno-suppressive drugs and ALS. Some attention has been given to reducing the lymphocyte count in the peripheral blood by passing it through an extracorporeal shunt and irradiating it outside the body. This method although tried so far only on a small scale and with a limited degree of success may perhaps, with development, become of value in the future. The drugs prednisone and Imuran (azathioprine) in combination are widely used and for immunosuppression are often given together with ALS. These substances in high dosage are toxic but haemodialysis before operation and during rejection crises reduces their toxicity in renal transplant cases.

Any of these regimes clearly carries with it the considerable risk of infection and the commonest cause of death after kidney grafting is not graft rejection but infection with fungi, viruses and bacteria. Another apparent complication noted in the last few years is the small but significant increase in reticulosarcomata following prolonged immunosuppressive therapy. This could conceivably be due to inhibition of the immunological surveillance mechanism (Chap. 11).

Anti-lymphocyte serum has the advantage of primarily affecting the thymus-dependent lymphocytes of the spleen and lymph nodes, and lymphocytes circulating in the blood. This results in a suppression of the cell-mediated immune response with only a slight effect on the circulating antibody response. Thus, whilst suppressing the graft rejection mechanisms ALS leaves the animal able to produce circulating antibody against infecting microorganisms and their products. However, infections caused by intracellular agents such as virus in which protection depends on cell-mediated immunity (p. 97) still remain a possible complication in this form of immunosuppression and different preparations of ALS may vary in their effect on the antibody response. Furthermore, ALS can destroy platelets because of shared platelet and leucocyte antigen and may require prior absorption with platelet suspensions. Anaphylactic reactions may occur because of the foreign nature of the protein and severe pain frequently occurs at the injection site.

The possibility arises that in the future the immune response to histocompatibility antigens may conceivably be prevented by giving passive antibody against the transplantation antigens in the same way as can rhesus immunization (p. 121).

FURTHER READING

Berenbaum, M. C. (1967). Transplantation and immunosuppression. In *Modern Trends in Immunology*, 2, p. 292. Ed. Cruickshank, R. & Weir, D. M. London: Butterworth.

James, K. (1967). Anti-lymphocyte antibody: a review. *Clin. exp. Immun.* **2,** 615.

Merrill, J. P. (1967). Human tissue transplantation. *Adv. Immun.* **2,** 615.

Porter, K. A. (1967). Symposium on tissue and organ transplantation. *J. clin. Path.,* Suppl. **20,** 415.

Rapaport, F. T. & Dausset, J. (1968). *Human Transplantation.* New York: Grune & Stratton.

Chapter 8

INFECTION, IMMUNITY AND PROTECTION

Earlier chapters of this book deal with the mechanisms and characteristics of acquired immunity, both cell-mediated and humoral, and with the interactions between antibody and antigen resulting for example in the lysis by complement of microorganisms. It is necessary however to stress that neither the production of antibody to the antigens of an invading microorganism, nor even the combination of the antibody with such antigen, is in itself any guarantee that the infective agent will be inactivated or eliminated from the body. Microorganisms have numerous ways of protecting themselves from, and sidetracking, the immune reactions of the host. For example, the pneumococcus secretes large quantities of capsular polysaccharide that repels phagocytes and mops up antibody as it is produced, thus allowing the pneumococcus itself to proliferate unhindered. Trypanosomes appear to change their surface antigenic make-up from one generation to the next, so that the antibody made in response to the antigens of the original organism is inactive against the second generation of organisms. Many microorganisms, particularly tubercle bacilli, brucellae and many viruses, disappear inside tissue cells before sufficient antibody is produced to act against them. It has in the last few years been found that leprosy bacilli, which are similar in many ways to tubercle bacilli, have the ability to destroy the cells in the thymus-dependent areas of the lymphoid tissues. This prevents the mounting of a cell-mediated immune response (p. 31) against the invading organisms and allows its unhindered proliferation. The same appears to be true for cutaneous leishmaniasis where instances have been described of a loss of cell-mediated immunity. In short, a particular microorganism is pathogenic because in some way it is able to circumvent, at least initially, the immune mechanisms of the host.

Immunity in Bacterial Infections

Antibody-mediated immunity

Antitoxins

Many microorganisms owe their pathogenic abilities to the production of exotoxins. Amongst diseases dependent on this type of mechanism are diphtheria, tetanus, gas gangrene and botulism. Antibodies either acquired by immunization, previous infection or given passively as antiserum are able to neutralize these bacterial toxins. To give protection, antibodies must either be present in sufficient quantity, as they would after administration of antiserum, or be produced faster than the toxin is produced by the microorganism. This would be likely to occur if the individual had previously been exposed to the organism or its products by natural infection or artificial immunization. In such a situation the infected individual would be able to mount a rapid secondary immune response (p. 27). The previously exposed individual can be said to have an 'immunological memory' of the toxin, having a population of cells ready and waiting to respond rapidly to the slightest whiff of the exotoxin. The infected individual with no 'immunological memory' may require to be given antibody prophylactically in order to tide him over the first stages of infection.

Bacterial toxins have been largely identified as enzymatic in nature and the antibody in some way is able to interfere with the ability of the enzyme to interact with its substrate. The antibody is not thought likely to interact with the active site of the enzyme but the nearer it reacts to this the more effective is its neutralizing power likely to be. The most probable explanation of the inhibitory effect of antibody is that it produces what is called 'steric hindrance', which simply means that it gets in the way and physically prevents the enzyme from coming in close apposition to its substrate (Fig. 22). To support this idea is the finding that antibody is much more effective against enzymes which have high molecular weight substrates than it is against those with low molecular weight substrates. Figure 22 shows how such a low molecular weight substance can still come in contact with the active site of the enzyme even in the presence of antibody.

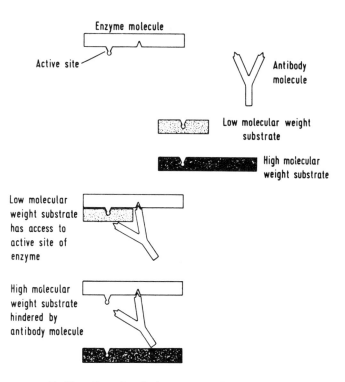

Blocking effect of antibody to enzyme substrate is effective only if enzyme substrate is of high molecular weight.

Fig. 22 Diagrammatic view of the possible 'steric hindrance' effect of antibody against an enzyme toxin. A low molecular weight substrate avoids the blocking effect of the antibody molecule. The closer the antibody is attached to the active site of the enzyme the more effective will be its blocking action.

In the case where a microorganism does not secrete exotoxins, the protection afforded by antibodies depends on the direct effect of antibodies attached to the surface of the microorganism. This can have a number of effects the most important of which is in encouraging phagocytosis by macrophages of the blood (monocytes) or the polymorphonuclear leucocytes. The antibody in some way, perhaps by altering the surface charge, changes the surface characteristics of the microorganism so making it more susceptible to phagocytosis. The phagocytic cell in many instances can then digest the microorganism by secreting into the phagocytic vacuole a variety of digestive enzymes carried in the intracellular lysozomes. However, some microorganisms such as the streptococci and *Mycobacterium tuberculosis,* are able to resist intracellular digestion. The streptococcus carries, as part of its cell wall, a substance known as M protein, which confers the ability to resist digestion by the enzymes. If immunity exists to the M protein, by previous exposure or artificial immunization, the streptococcus is susceptible to intracellular digestion. Rough (avirulent) strains of salmonella are susceptible to intracellular digestion whilst the smooth (virulent) strains are able to resist digestion in some way. In the case of enteric infections such as those due to *Salmonella typhi* or *Vibrio cholerae,* antibodies can be secreted into the intestinal lumen and attack the organism before it invades the intestinal mucosa. These antibodies secreted by an immune individual are known as copro-antibodies and may be predominantly IgA in type. The IgA immunoglobulin is selectively produced in intestinal and respiratory mucous membranes (p. 48). Other effects of antibody reacting with the surface of the microorganism are cell lysis, brought about by the activation of the complement system, and simple localization of the organism by agglutination or clumping.

It is even conceivable that antibody acts by coating growing bacteria so that their daughter cells, when formed, remain in a clump instead of dispersing. Attachment of bacteria to the host's red blood cells in the presence of antibody and complement is another way in which phagocytosis is encouraged. This phenomenon is known as *immune adherence* but as yet it is not clear exactly how the attachment to red cells takes place.

Apart from the clumping effect on the bacteria, agglutination seems to have little effect on the viability or respiratory activity of the organisms although it is conceivable that the bacteria at the centre of a large mass of clumped organisms would be limited in their metabolic activity simply by a lack of sufficient nutrient material.

Precipitation of antibody on the surface of certain parasitic nematodes has been proposed as a mechanism whereby the excretory orifices of the worm are blocked, thus interfering with its metabolism.

Acquired cellular immunity

Macrophage-dependent cellular immunity

The inter-relations of antibody-mediated immune mechanisms and acquired cellular immunity are not yet clearly defined. It is known, however, that macrophages from animals immune to tubercle bacilli are more actively phagocytic than those taken from a normal animal. Enhancement of cellular immunity has been reported with macrophages from brucella-infected animals; such cells restricted the intracellular growth of brucellae although the enhancement was dependent on the initial immunization with a living virulent strain of the organism. The same phenomenon has been found after *Listeria monocytogenes* infection in mice where macrophages isolated from the peritoneal cavity acquire an increased resistance to listeria and at the same time an increased intracellular resistance to tubercle bacilli and brucellae. This increased resistance is non-specific in the immunological sense in that the enhanced activity of the macrophage is directed not only at the species of organism responsible for the initial infection but also at other species.

The non-specific enhancement of macrophage activity, including their ability to kill microorganisms and spread themselves throughout the peritoneal cavity to mop up an infectious agent, appears to depend partly upon the transfer of an as yet undefined stimulus from lymphoid cells which have reacted immunologically to the initial injection of microorganisms. Thus the first part of the response depends on a specific immune reaction on the part of lymphoid cells to an agent such as *L. monocytogenes*; these cells proliferate and in turn activate the macrophages so that not only do they handle listeria more effectively but also other bacterial agents. This phenomenon can be shown quite clearly by transferring stimulated mouse lymphoid cells to an unstimulated recipient; the recipient's macrophages then assume these enhanced bactericidal and spreading properties.

Immunity in Virus Infections

Antibody-mediated immunity

Blood stream or surface protection

In virus infections the efficiency of antibody depends largely on whether the virus passes through the blood stream in order to reach its target organ. A well known example of a virus which follows such a route is the polio virus; this crosses the intestinal wall, enters the blood stream and passes to the spinal cord and brain where it proliferates. Small amounts of antibody in the blood can neutralize the virus before it reaches its target cells in the nervous system. A number of other viruses behave in the same way and pass through the blood stream on their way to their target organ; examples are the viruses of measles, mumps, rubella and chickenpox. Disease caused by these viruses is characterized by a prolonged incubation period. In comparison, in another group of virus diseases with a short incubation period such as influenza and the common cold, the viruses do not pass through the blood stream, as their target organ is their site of entry to the body, namely the respiratory mucous membranes. In this type of infection, even a high blood level of antibody will be relatively ineffective against these viruses in comparison with its effect on the blood-borne viruses. For this antibody to act on such respiratory viruses it must pass through the mucous membranes into the respiratory secretion. Examination of the antibody content of mucous secretion has shown that in contrast to the blood there is very little IgG antibody and often no IgM and it thus appears that the mucous membranes are not very permeable to antibodies of these classes. However it has been found that the predominant immunoglobulin in these secretions is IgA manufactured by plasma cells in the lamina propria of the mucous membranes. IgA present in nasal secretions has been shown to be responsible for most of the neutralizing activity against common cold viruses. One conclusion which can be drawn from this is that conventional immunization methods designed to produce high blood levels of antibody are unlikely to be effective against viruses which attack the mucous membranes, and some effort is being directed at developing methods for stimulating local antibody production of IgA type in the mucous membranes themselves. An example of this is the intranasal administration of a live attenuated influenza virus which has been used extensively in the United States and the Soviet Union. The high degree of immunity provided by the oral polio vaccine seems likely in part to be due to locally produced antibody in the gut neutralizing the virus even before it reaches the blood stream. The presence of IgA antibody against polio virus has recently been demonstrated in the faeces, in duodenal fluid and in saliva. In contrast, after injection of inactivated virus vaccine no such antibodies could be found. The nasopharyngeal antibodies have been shown to persist for at least 300 days which is consistent with the long term protection which the oral vaccine affords. It is of some interest that the levels of IgA antipolio antibody were found to be lower in children who had their tonsils and adenoids removed. Furthermore primary vaccination in such children produced lower levels of these specific antibodies than in children who had not had their tonsils removed.

Persistence of virus and 'antigenic drift'

One of the major differences between viral and bacterial immunity is that the former is usually of much longer duration and in many instances lifelong, e.g. in measles and mumps. An explanation of this may be that some virus remains within tissue cells and is protected from immune rejection. Occasionally some virus material is released and thus maintains a persisting level of immunity. The possibility exists that such virus antigen will combine with antibody resulting in the formation of toxic complexes with ensuing hypersensitivity of type 3 (p. 77). The existence of such a phenomenon could have considerable importance in the pathogenesis of some viral diseases. In those virus infections in which repeated attacks occur, e.g. influenza and the common cold, fresh infection is due to different strains of the virus which are relatively insusceptible to the antibodies induced by previous infection by other strains.

Influenza epidemics have occurred at 2–3 year intervals over the last 40 years and type B virus outbreaks tend to alternate with type A epidemics. The main viral antigen responsible for inducing immunity is the haemagglutinin (HA). Influenza viruses types A and B have different HA antigens and within these two types there are a number of distinct families with HA antigens which differ markedly from one another. In type A infection, the families A, A_0, A_1 and A_2 have appeared successively, and each in turn has dominated the epidemic history of influenza for periods of 10–15 years and is then displaced by later antigenic variants. It is believed that this 'antigenic drift' from one virus family to another is one of progressive mutation, and that immunity against earlier strains becomes obsolete once further antigenic variants have appeared.

Cell-mediated immunity

The humoral immune response is probably the predominant form of immunity responsible for protection from reinfection by viruses. For this reason immunization procedures aim at producing circulating or mucous membrane antibody. In the case of primary virus infections the position is not very clear but it seems likely to involve some form of cell-mediated immunity. It is known that children with congenital hypogammaglobulin-aemia (p. 65) can recover from virus infections without producing any virus-neutralizing antibody. Although it is possible that these children are producing small amounts of neutralizing anti-body sufficient to provide immunity, it is significant that the capacity to resist virus infection is associated with normal cell-mediated immune reactions. These subjects are able to develop normal delayed hypersensitivity reactions to bacterial and viral antigens and contact sensitivity to simple chemicals (p. 80). In patients with Swiss-type agammaglobulinaemia (p. 66), who have an additional cell-mediated immune deficiency, sus-ceptibility to virus infection is very great and death often follows the development of severe generalized vaccinia after routine inoculation of live vaccine.

Further evidence that cell-mediated immune reactions are involved in resistance to viruses comes from the finding that, just as in the case of intracellular bacterial agents such as tubercle bacilli and brucellae, cell-mediated reactions of the delayed hypersensitivity type (p. 78) can be demonstrated after many types of virus infection. The best known example of this is the reaction soon after revaccination with vaccinia virus where there is an accelerated reaction (compared to primary vaccination) reaching its maximum at 72 hours with a minimum of tissue damage and a rapid elimination of the infective agent.

Babies with congenital rubella infection have been shown to excrete virus for periods up to 18 months of age. Such infants can be shown to possess high levels of IgM anti-rubella antibody which indicates that they have not developed neonatal tolerance (p. 50) to the virus. Their cell-mediated immune mechanisms seem, however, to be defective due to a direct effect of the virus on lymphocytes. Lymphocytes taken from such an infant do not respond normally to the plant mitogen PHA (p. 32) and normal leucocytes infected *in vitro* with the virus can be shown to become defective in the same way. Depression of lymphocyte reactivity has been associated with a number of virus infections, e.g. rubella, herpes, Newcastle disease virus (causing fowl pest) and hepatitis virus. This effect on lymphocytes seems likely to affect the pathogenesis of virus infections.

Interferon

A quite distinct type of resistance mechanism in virus infection is the production by the infected host cells of a substance known as 'interferon'. This material interferes with the synthesis of new virus by tissue cells of the host. Interferon, unlike antibody, is not specific for the virus which may have induced its formation but is able to interfere with other quite different species of virus. Interferon probably plays a very important role in eliminating virus in non-immune individuals and the rise in level of interferon appears to coincide with the phase of virus elimination whilst circulating antibody levels are found to rise subsequent to this.

Immunity to Protozoa and Helminths

The life cycles of organisms in this category are complicated and the immune response to be effective has to interrupt the cycle at a stage when the parasite is accessible to the immune processes.

Protozoa

Malaria infections are initiated by sporozoites which transform into exoerythrocytic schizonts in the liver, and at this stage there is recognizable immunity. The schizonts rupture and discharge their merozoites into the peripheral circulation where they invade erythrocytes. There appears at this stage to be an alteration in the permeability of the red cell membrane so that immunoglobulin molecules can enter and attack the parasite. Antibodies are readily detectable in the serum and increase until the crisis 7–10 days later and then slowly decline. Because these antibodies are able to get access to the parasite only during a relatively short period of its life cycle, immunity is incomplete and the host usually fails to eliminate the parasite completely.

This state in which the organisms persist in small numbers in the tissues in the presence of an immune reaction is called *premunition* by parasitologists.

The efficacy of the immune mechanisms against trypanosomes is complicated by the fact that the parasites can change their surface antigenic constitution from one generation to the next. The number of variants which can be produced by a single strain is at least 20. It is not yet clear how the organism controls the generation of the variants, but variation is thought to arise by selection of mutants from a heterogeneous population of parasites.

This complication means that the immune response has great difficulty in keeping up with the antigenic changes in the parasite, and in the case of the trypanosomes responsible for African sleeping sickness the parasite does not induce an effective immunity, the infected subject developing a progressive infection with invasion of the central nervous system leading to death. Trypanosomiasis is associated with high levels of IgM immunoglobulins in both the blood and CSF. It is not certain if this is due to the repeated new antigenic stimuli resulting from changes in the organism or if the parasite in some way influences directly the cells of the immune system. Increased immunoglobulin production is a common finding in protozoal infections and often affects all classes of immunoglobulins. Because usually less than 5 per cent of the total immunoglobulin appears to react specifically with the inducing parasite it is probable that protozoa stimulate the lymphoid cells in a non-specific way to overproduce immunoglobulins.

Helminths

Helminths like protozoa go through a complex life cycle and protective immune mechanisms appear to act only at an early stage in the cycle. The main stimulus appears to be due to antigens derived from the adult worm and the immunity derived from this acts on new parasites entering the body. A noteworthy feature of these infections is the appearance of IgE (reaginic) antibodies (p. 72) with pulmonary oesinophilia, and it seems likely that immediate hypersensitivity reactions of the anaphylactic type (type 1) are involved in the pathogenesis of helminth infection. Migration of larvae into the lungs is sometimes associated with eosinophil infiltration and pneumonia which can be fatal.

Saprophytic Fungi and Respiratory Disease

Allergic alveolitis and anaphylaxis

A few examples of pulmonary hypersensitivity to inhaled fungal antigens have been reported in the last few years. The existence of a state of immunity has been confirmed by the finding of precipitating antibodies in the serum. The first of these disorders to be recognized was farmers' lung disease in which precipitating antibodies could be demonstrated against antigens derived from mouldy hay. The antigen has since been found to be *Microspora faeni*. Subsequently precipitins have been demonstrated against *Aspergillus clavatus* in maltworkers exposed to high concentrations of *A. clavatus* spores from contaminated barley and against *Coniosporium corticale* in the serum of maple bark strippers. It is likely that following exposure to high concentrations of any of a variety of fungal spores individuals would produce precipitating antibodies and thus this form of pulmonary hypersensitivity may be more widespread than has so far been identified. The hypersensitivity reaction induced by the presence of precipitating antibodies would be of the toxic-complex (type 3) form inducing a diffuse pulmonary interstitial pneumonitis which has been termed allergic alveolitis. Some of the antigens responsible for this form of hypersensitivity can also provoke in susceptible individuals the anaphylactic (type 1) response exemplified by pulmonary asthma.

Common Vaccination Procedures

Efficacy and hazards

It is generally accepted that one effective way of controlling the spread of infectious disease is by immunization with antigens derived from the appropriate organism. The isolation and bulk preparation of the particular antigens which confer protective immunity is a major difficulty, but success in this field with a number of potentially dangerous microorganisms has radically altered the chances of them causing widespread disease in the population. The use of diphtheria toxoid (inactivated diphtheria toxin) is a noteworthy example. In Scotland, notifications of diphtheria averaged about 10,000 cases annually before 1940 when widespread immunization was instituted. The incidence of the disease rapidly decreased thereafter and with the exception of an outbreak in 1968, involving six cases none of whom had been fully immunized, the disease can be said to have been virtually eradicated. Much consideration has been given to the safety of vaccines and it is generally agreed that the greatest danger arises from the introduction of infection at the time of administration of the vaccine. Complications such as encephalitis after smallpox vaccination, febrile convulsions after whooping-cough vaccination and neurological complication after rabies vaccination are extremely rare phenomena and the risk is by far outweighed by the protection that immunization can give from the disease itself.

Antigens of Microorganisms

Bacterial and viral antigens are in common use in medical practice as a means of inducing immunity to infectious diseases such as smallpox, diphtheria, measles, poliomyelitis, typhoid fever and many others. There are four main types of antigen preparations or *vaccines*.

1. *Toxoids* are the soluble exotoxins of bacteria such as diphtheria and tetanus bacilli, which have been modified and rendered less toxic by the addition of formalin or gentle heating. They are administered either in solution or precipitated on alum. Many years of useful immunity can be achieved by these procedures.

2. *Killed vaccines* are cultured organisms killed by heat, usually 60°C for 1 hour, ultraviolet irradiation or chemicals such as phenol, alcohol or formalin. Protection against whooping cough, poliomyelitis and perhaps cholera can be achieved in this way.

3. *Antigens isolated from infectious agents,* for example the capsular polysaccharide of the pneumococci. A diffusible factor of *B. anthracis* and a cell wall preparation of haemolytic streptococci have been shown to induce immunity, but such preparations are not in general use in medical practice.

4. *Attenuated living vaccines* are made from strains of organisms that have lost their virulence by growth in culture (e.g. Pasteur's chicken cholera vaccine, p. 1) or in animals when the conditions are not favourable for the growth and proliferation of the virulent strain. Strains emerge which, whilst not able to produce disease, can induce immunity; such strains are known as *attenuated* organisms. The BCG vaccine (Bacille Calmette-Guérin) is the outstanding example of this type of vaccine, providing protection against tuberculosis in man. The oral administration of a strain of poliomyelitis virus induces a powerful immunity without producing the disease. The virus spreads from one individual to another and so is able to produce immunity in a community. An attenuated strain of yellow fever virus has been developed, obtained from the original virulent material by prolonged cultivation in tissue culture. Attenuated strains of measles virus are also used.

Routine procedures

The determining factors in the selection of immunization procedures for a particular population must depend on local environmental conditions and epidemiological considerations. In Britain, a child is immunized during its first year of life with a vaccine containing diphtheria and tetanus toxoids in combination with a killed suspension of whooping-cough (*Bordetella pertussis*) organisms. This is known as triple vaccine and its efficacy as an immunizing agent is in part due to the adjuvant effect of the pertussis component. This procedure is repeated on two further occasions and at the same time oral polio vaccine is usually given. Vaccination against smallpox is achieved by giving one dose of the vaccinia vaccine during the second year when the

Age	Prophylactic	Interval	Notes
During the first year of life	Diph/Tet/Pert and oral Polio vaccine. (First dose)		The earliest age at which the first dose should be given is 3 months, but a better general immunological response can be expected if the first dose is delayed to 6 months of age
	Diph/Tet/Pert and oral Polio vaccine. (Second dose)	Preferably after an interval of 6–8 weeks	
	Diph/Tet/Pert and oral Polio vaccine. (Third dose)	Preferably after an interval of 6 months	
During the second year of life	Measles vaccination		While the second year is recommended for routine vaccination against smallpox in special circumstances it may be carried out during the first year
	Smallpox vaccination		With the exception of smallpox revaccination these may be given, if desired at 3 years of age to children entering nursery schools, attending day nurseries or living in children's homes
At 5 years of age or school entry	Diph/Tet and oral Polio vaccine or		
	Diph/Tet/Polio vaccine Smallpox revaccination		
Between 10 and 13 years of age	BCG vaccine		For tuberculin-negative children
At 15–19 years of age or on leaving school	Polio vaccine (oral or inactivated). Tetanus toxoid. Smallpox revaccination		

chances of developing complications appear to be much decreased. Booster doses of all these vaccines are usually given at 5 years of age and tetanus, polio and smallpox again at age 15–19. Table 5 shows the recommended Schedules of the Department of Health and Social Security.

FURTHER READING

Evans, D. G. (1969). Immunization against infectious diseases. *Br. med. Bull.* **25,** No. 2.

Gell, P. G. H. & Coombs, R. R. A. (1968). Immunoprophylaxis and immunotherapy. In *Clinical Aspects of Immunology*, 2nd ed., Sect. V. Oxford: Blackwell.

Hobson, D. (1967). Immunization against respiratory virus infection. In *Modern Trends in Immunology*, 2, p. 53. Ed. Cruickshank, R. & Weir, D. M. London: Butterworth.

Wright, G. P. (1968). Protective immunity. In *Clinical Aspects of Immunology*, 2nd ed. Ed. Gell, P. G. H. & Coombs, R. R. A. Oxford: Blackwell.

Chapter 9

AUTOIMMUNITY

A fundamental characteristic of an animal's immune system is that it does not under normal circumstances react against its own body constituents. There exists a mechanism which enables the cells of the immune system to recognize what is 'foreign' and what is 'self'. Attempts to explain the absence of reactions against self go back to the early days of immunology when Paul Ehrlich enunciated his well known doctrine of 'horror auto-toxicus'. Ehrlich and Morgenroth in 1900 after immunizing a goat with red blood cells of other goats found that although the animal readily made antibodies against the red cells of other goats these antibodies failed to react with the animal's own red cells. It was thus clear that in some way the immunological response to self antigens was prevented. So powerful was the influence of Paul Ehrlich that it seemed inconceivable that in any circumstances the rule could be broken so that an immunological reaction against self could develop. This view continued to be held despite clinical evidence indicating that diseases existed in which the patient was apparently destroying his own cells.

The main reason that observations of this type failed to achieve the recognition they deserved was the absence of sero-logical techniques capable of demonstrating convincingly the existence of antibodies able to react with tissue cells or of the presence of such antibodies actually attached to cells. It was not until 1945 that immunologists were provided with this vital tool, when Coombs, Mourant and Race described a technique which detected the presence of antibody globulin on red blood cells by the simple expedient of adding an antiserum against human globulin which, after reacting with the globulin coating the cells, linked the cells together and agglutinated them. This method was particularly valuable for showing antibody globulin adsorbed to cells which was in itself unable to agglutinate the cells. This technique is commonly known as the 'Coombs' or 'antiglobulin' test (p. 141). The development of the antiglobulin techniques led to the use of antiglobulin sera in a variety of different ways many of which involved complicated technical operations but which essentially were based on the original antiglobulin method. Amongst the most important of the developments of the method is the fluorescent antibody technique in which one of the most commonly used procedures is to label an antiglobulin serum with a fluorescent marker (fluorescein isothiocyanate) so that the reaction of the labelled antiglobulin with, for example, globulin-coated cells can be visualized under UV light microscopy. Under these conditions the sites of attachment of the fluorescein-labelled antiglobulin show up as bright apple-green fluorescent areas (p. 144).

The recognition of autoimmune disease

These methods allowed a breakthrough in the recognition of a variety of human and animal diseases in which antibodies could be convincingly demonstrated in serum capable of reacting with a number of different antigens of the individual's own tissues.

The first of these was the demonstration that in some types of haemolytic anaemia in man the red blood cells were coated with antibody globulin. This was soon followed by the finding of an autoantibody serum factor in the blood of patients with a severe connective tissue disease called systemic lupus erythematosus (SLE). This factor appeared to be antibody against the nuclei of tissue cells and was called anti-nuclear factor (ANF). At the same time workers interested in diseases of the thyroid gland demonstrated the presence of an antibody to thyroglobulin in patients with a particular form of interstitial thyroiditis known as Hashimoto's disease.

The first recognizable clinical description of acquired haemolytic anaemia was given in 1898 in France, and in 1908 haemolytic activity against red cells was found in the serum of patients in whom intense haemolysis was taking place *in vivo*. These early observations were neglected until 30 years later when Damashek and Schwartz again reported haemolysins in patients suffering from haemolytic anaemia, and with the introduction of the Coombs test in 1945 the immunological basis of the disease was put on a firm foundation.

Associated with the accumulating evidence on the autoimmune nature of the haemolysins in acute haemolytic anaemia, there arose the need to consider the meaning of foreignness and self-recognition and the mechanisms underlying the ability of the body to differentiate between 'self' and 'non-self'. A solution to the problem this created in immunological theory was offered by Burnet and Fenner in 1949. At that time antibody production was envisaged in terms of the antigen acting as a template for modifying the globulin molecules to a form which was complementary to that of antigen (p. 54). It was considered that antigen might act either on the already formed protein chain and bring about a reconfiguration of the chain, or that the antigen induced a chemical rearrangement of the globulin molecule as it was formed. Burnet and Fenner, whilst accepting this direct template theory, included the notion of 'self-markers' attached to body components by which antibody-forming cells were able to recognize them, thus rendering them immunologically inert. They also predicted that an equivalent tolerance to foreign antigens should be demonstrable if these had been introduced at an appropriate stage in embryonic life, while the animal's immune system was in the process of learning to recognize the 'self-markers' of its own tissues. This prediction was later confirmed experimentally by Medawar and his colleagues who showed that if neonatal mice were injected with transplantation antigen from another strain of mice, they would later be able to accept skin grafts which an animal not injected neonatally would rapidly reject. Burnet soon followed his 'self-marker' theory by his rather more plausible 'clonal selection' theory. This allowed the antigen no part in impressing a pattern on the antibody-producing cells. The capacity to produce a given antibody was regarded as a genetically determined quality of certain clones or families of mesenchymal cells, the function of the antigen being to stimulate cells of these clones to proliferation and antibody production. The theory postulated that in the early stages of embryonic development, mutation of cells led to a variety of random arrangements in the globulin molecules so that a very large number of clones were generated which could correspond to potential antigenic determinants (p. 54). To explain the inability of the antibody-forming system to react with self,

Burnet proposed that the immature cells could be destroyed if they came across the antigens with which they could react at this early stage. Whenever the antigenic determinants were freely present in the body and accessible to the corresponding immunologically competent cells, such destructive contacts would be inevitable. Tolerance would result from the elimination or inhibition of all cell clones which had the ability to react with antigenic determinants present in the body. After birth when foreign antigen entered the tissues antibody to it would be produced by specific stimulation of those cells in clones pre-adapted to react with the corresponding antigenic determinants. On the basis of this theory Burnet accounted for the development of autoimmune disease as a failure of the maintenance of the non-self-reactive population of antibody-forming cells (see also p. 54).

Possible mechanism involved in the development of autoimmunity

The question now arises of how the normal controlling mechanism fails with the resulting inability to maintain self-recognition manifested by immune reactions against self.

Table 6 Mechanisms of autoantibody formation

1. EVASION of normal tolerance to 'self' antigens
    (a) Hidden antigens
    (b) Altered antigens –
           chemicals, drugs, infectious agents

2. BREAKDOWN of tolerance mechanism
    (a) Agents affecting antibody forming cells –
           chemicals, drugs, infectious agents
    (b) Genetically determined lack of efficiency of tolerance control mechanisms

There are two main ways (Table 6) in which this tolerance-maintaining mechanism could conceivably be overcome. The first involves evasion or circumvention of a normally functioning mechanism and the second failure of the mechanism itself.

In the first category evasion may occur in two possible ways: (1) because a particular body antigen is not accessible to the cells of the immune system as the antigen is hidden within a cell or tissue – these antigens are known as sequestered antigens; (2) because a tissue antigen is altered in some way by a chemical agent, a drug or an infectious agent.

Sequestered antigens

Hidden or sequestered antigens do seem to exist and the best examples of these are sperm antigens and lens antigen of the eye. Sperm can be shown to acquire an antigen during maturation which is absent from the immature germinal cells and antibodies can be induced in the guinea-pig by immunizing with autologous sperm showing that the immune system fails to recognize the sperm as part of self. Orchitis can be induced by combining the sperm with an adjuvant which gives a boost to the immune response and at the same time in some way allows the stimulated lymphoid cells and antibody to gain access to the sperm-forming tissues. Orchitis in man is a rare complication of mumps infection in which it is assumed that the virus damages the basement membrane barrier of the seminiferous tubules and the cells of the immune system are thus allowed entry and initiate an immune response.

In the case of the lens it can be shown that if a rabbit is injected with bovine lens material, it develops antibodies which react with its own lens *in vitro*. Occasionally the surgical extraction of a lens for cataract is succeeded by inflammatory changes in retained lens substance sometimes affecting the other unoperated lens, and the same phenomenon can be induced experimentally in animals.

Interpretations of observations of this type is fraught with complications and can be regarded at present only as speculative evidence to support the concept of sequestered antigens as an initiating factor in autoimmune disease.

Altered antigens

Evidence in support of the second proposed way in which normal tolerance mechanisms are circumvented is more concrete. Experimental studies of tolerance evasion by altered antigens have been carried out with purified proteins, conjugates of hapten and protein, and with cellular antigens. Some of the most definitive work is that carried out in America by Weigle who showed that rabbits made tolerant to bovine serum albumen (BSA) and then immunized with the cross-reacting antigen human serum albumen (HSA) eventually made antibodies which could react with BSA. The same result was obtained with chemically modified BSA. A closer approximation to auto-immune disease is provided by experiments using thyroglobulin in rabbits; not only are anti-rabbit thyroglobulin antibodies induced by injection of altered thyroglobulin but inflammatory lesions are also found in their thyroid glands.

Shared antigens

There has been considerable interest in the last few years in the role of microorganisms as a source of cross-reacting antigens sharing antigenic determinants with tissue components. The ability of viruses to bring about alterations of cell membranes has been suggested by studies on the effect of herpes and rabies viruses on tissue culture cells. New cell surface antigens, which appear to act as transplantation antigens, have been found in mouse cells infected with herpes and also with polyoma viruses.

There is an antigen in human colon extractable even from sterile foetal human colon, which is similar to a polysaccharide antigen present in *E. coli* 014. It is conceivable that the inflammatory condition of the colon known as ulcerative colitis, in which anti-colon antibodies are found, is due to an immune reaction initiated by the cross-reacting bacterial antigen. Similarly the Group A streptococci, which are closely associated with rheumatic fever, have an antigen in common with a human heart antigen. Heart lesions are a common finding in rheumatic fever and anti-heart antibody is found in just over 50 per cent of patients with the condition.

Nephritogenic strains of Type 12 Group A streptococci carry surface antigens similar to those found in human glomeruli and infection by these organisms has been associated with the development of acute nephritis.

Drugs as haptens

Drugs can act as haptens (p. 15) which bind to tissue proteins. The resulting complex may be antigenic and result in an immune reaction which damages cells coated with the drug. An example

110

of this is a metabolic breakdown product of the drug α-methyldopa (used in the treatment of hypertension). The immune response generated by these drug-altered cells can then result in haemolysis of the affected cells and α-methyldopa is thought to have the effect of altering or exposing normally hidden red cell antigens. The antibody which results has been found to combine with Rhesus antigens present on the surface of the patient's own normal erythrocytes. One hypothesis is that the α-methyldopa is incorporated into the Rhesus antigen when the red cell is being made and the change this induces prevents the antigen being recognized as self. (See also discussion of the effects of the drug Sedormid, p. 76.)

Disturbed immunological mechanisms

The second main category of mechanisms by means of which autoimmune reactions may develop (Table 6) are those due to alteration in the cellular processes on which maintenance of normal tolerance depends. One way in which this might occur is by the direct effect of a chemical, a drug or an infectious agent on the lymphoid tissues. Alternatively, it is conceivable that the loss of normal tolerance control might be due to an inherited defect or lack of efficiency in the lymphoid cell population.

There is much speculation amongst immunologists and clinicians on the role of infectious agents acting *directly* on the lymphoid tissues as a cause of autoimmune disease. This stems from the experimental evidence on the induction of autoimmune disease using tissue antigens combined with Freund's complete adjuvant. This water-in-oil emulsion owes its powerful stimulating effect on the lymphoid tissues, to killed mycobacteria which are incorporated in the oil. Without the mycobacterial component, tissue antigens are much less effective in disturbing the tolerance mechanisms. Rabbits injected with *Mycobacterium tuberculosis* alone have been shown to develop autoantibodies against a wide range of autologous tissues. The same phenomenon is found in a number of chronic infections in the human such as syphilis, actinomycosis and chronic tuberculosis. Infection with *Mycoplasma pneumoniae*, responsible for a disease known as primary atypical pneumonia, is associated with the development of IgM agglutinins in the patient's serum, which in the cold will react with the patient's own red cells.

111

A leukaemia virus has in the last few years been found in a strain of mice (New Zealand Black or NZB mice) characterized by the early development of autoimmune disease including auto-immune haemolytic anaemia and immune complex nephritis. The virus has been found in many body tissues and in the blood and can be seen in lymphoid organs, attached to the surface of lymphocytes. Similar virus particles have been found in embryos of the NZB strain, suggesting that it is passed through the placenta or is associated with the germ cells. The association of the virus with lymphocyte membranes has attracted the attention of immunologists and there has been speculation that the presence of the virus might interfere with normal lymphocyte reactivity to antigens. It is known (p. 50) that antigens can react with the lymphocyte surface and that this is probably one stimulus to immune transformation of these cells. The virus could conceivably upset the mechanisms controlling lymphocyte reactivity so that they respond abnormally to antigens to which they should remain tolerant. This idea receives some support from experiments in which animals stimulated with certain microorganisms (e.g. tubercle bacilli or corynebacteria) or the products of organisms (e.g. bacterial endotoxin) do not develop the expected immune tolerance when these antigens are administered in a way which would induce tolerance in normal animals.

The Pathogenesis of Autoimmune Disease

There is even more uncertainty in this area than exists with respect to the underlying abnormalities and stimuli which induce the autoimmune response.

Autoimmune diseases can be classified as hypersensitivity reactions on the basis of the definitions given in Chapter 6. These immune reactions, in contrast to those involved in protection from infectious disease, actually bring about severe and some-times fatal reactions affecting the individual's own tissues and cells. The hypersensitivity reactions are divided into four types and three of these encompass autoimmune reactions.

Cytolytic or cytotoxic (type 2) reactions

The foremost of the autoimmune conditions in this category is autoimmune haemolytic anaemia. Here the antibodies are of two main types: (1) antibodies of the IgM class which agglutinate the patient's own red cells in the cold; (2) antibodies of the IgG class which do not usually bring about direct agglutination of the red cells but can be detected by the Coombs test (p. 141) using an antiglobulin serum.

The anaemia is caused largely by the removal of antibody-coated cells in the spleen or the liver. Only rarely does lysis or agglutination take place to any extent in the circulation and involve the uptake of serum complement. Whilst normal red cells survive with a half life in the circulation of just over three weeks, in this form of anaemia they are unlikely to have a half life of more than one week.

Other forms of haemolytic anaemia exist including drug-induced types and those involving infective agents such as mycoplasma. Drugs involved include penicillin, phenacetin, quinine and α methyldopa. The anaemia is brought about by the reaction of antibody with the drug linked as a hapten to the red cell surface resulting in haemolysis. The precise details of the haptenic groups responsible for antigenic stimulation and their linkage to the red cell surface are uncertain. In mycoplasma infections the IgM cold agglutinins react with a widely distributed red cell antigen known as the I antigen.

Drug-induced agranulocytosis and thrombocytopoenia have also been described in which the leucocytes or platelets are destroyed by antibody directed at a complex of the drug and cell surface structures. Sedormid purpura has already been mentioned (p. 76).

Toxic-complex (type 3) reactions

Complexes of antibody and tissue antigens, particularly nuclear antigens, are the cause of glomerulonephritis in a number of autoimmune states and notably in a disease known as systemic lupus erythematosus where a wide range of anti-tissue antibodies is found, and in the similar type of disease of NZB mice. Complexes of antinuclear antibody and nuclear antigen, together with complement, can readily be demonstrated in the glomerular capillaries. The glomerular basement membranes become thickened and secondary changes develop in the renal tubules with progressive renal failure.

Cell-mediated (type 4) reactions

There is no doubt that in both man and experimental animals the development of a number of autoimmune states is paralleled by the finding of cell-mediated reactions of the delayed hypersensitivity type as demonstrated by skin tests using tissue antigens. Whether the diseases are actually caused by immune reactions mediated by lymphoid cells is a matter of conjecture. Support for the role of cells in the disease process comes from studies in an experimental autoimmune disease known as autoimmune allergic encephalomyelitis. This is brought about by immunization of animals with brain homogenate in Freund's complete adjuvant and paralysis follows demyelination of motor nerve fibres. The disease can be transferred in inbred strains of rats by the injection of lymphoid cells from affected animals to normal animals. The same type of transfer has been performed in autoimmune thyroiditis. In the latter condition it is proposed that the sensitized lymphocytes produce a surface injury to the cells of the thyroid acini and thus allows the cytotoxic antibody frequently present in the serum of affected subjects, to enter the cell and react with intracellular antigens.

That there may be an interaction between cell-mediated immunity and a humoral antibody is emphasized by work on autoimmune orchitis in guinea-pigs. Animals injected with a purified testis homogenate in Freund's complete adjuvant develop cell-mediated immunity (as shown by the development of delayed hypersensitivity on skin testing) but no circulating antibody or testicular lesion. When these animals are injected with anti-testis antibody (from a guinea-pig injected with testis homogenate in incomplete Freund's adjuvant, i.e. without tubercle bacilli) orchitis can be shown to develop. This interpretation is supported by the finding that anti-testis antibody enters the seminiferous tubules (as shown by the indirect fluorescent antibody method, p. 144) at the same time as cell-mediated immunity first appears.

Other Diseases Associated with Autoimmune States

There is a large reservoir of diseases in which some form of autoantibody has been found but where neither the stimulus for autoantibody formation nor the role, if any, of immune reactions has been elucidated.

Among these conditions is rheumatoid arthritis in which an IgM antibody called rheumatoid factor is present in the serum. This antibody is detected *in vitro* by its ability to agglutinate red cells or latex particles which have been coated with IgG globulin (p. 148). The rheumatoid factor does not appear to be directly involved in the pathogenesis of the disease and no satisfactory explanation has been offered to account for its pathogenesis. The possibility has been suggested that infective agents are involved such as mycoplasma or chronic infective bacterial agents, and there are reports of the isolation of such agents from rheumatoid joint arthritis in man and in a number of other species. One suggestion is that the infective agent may modify the lymphoid tissues so that there is a failure of the normal tolerance control mechanisms (p. 111). Experimental arthritis can be induced in rats by the injection of Freund's complete adjuvant containing killed tubercle bacilli. This is a polyarthritis with mononuclear cell infiltration similar to the arthritis found in a human illness known as Reiter's syndrome, the main features of which are urethritis and arthritis and which may occur in the presence of a mycoplasma infection.

Recent evidence suggests that there may be an IgG form of rheumatoid factor present in both the blood and joint fluid of rheumatoid patients as well as the IgM type and that injection of autologous purified IgG into previously unaffected joints can induce acute arthritis. Further evidence suggesting that an antigen-antibody reaction is taking place is provided by the low complement levels found in patients' joint fluid.

Antibodies as a Consequence of Tissue Damage

In considering the role of autoantibodies as a possible cause of autoimmune disease it should be remembered that antibodies of IgM type, directed at subcellular antigens, can be readily induced by various forms of tissue damage. These arise secondarily to the damage and appear to have no role in perpetuating it. Antibodies of this type can readily be induced in rats by the injection of the hepatotoxic agent carbon tetrachloride, and it was subsequently found that normal rats, mice and hamsters have some IgM anti-tissue antibody in their serum. A possible physiological role for these antibodies is suggested by the finding *in vitro* of a chemotactic effect on rat polymorphs of a mixture of the antitissue antibody and its antigen. Thus the antibody might be responsible for initiating a phagocytic cell clearing process to deal with the breakdown products of normal cell turnover. All autoantibodies are therefore not necessarily autoaggressive although the history of immunity and protection inculcates the idea of antibodies acting solely as aggressive agents.

FURTHER READING

Asherson, G. L. (1968). The role of micro-organisms in auto-immune responses. *Progr. Allergy.* **12,** 192.

Asherson, G. L. (1968). Auto-antibody production as a breakdown of immune tolerance. In *Regulation of the Antibody Response,* p. 68. Ed. Cinader, B. Springfield, Illinois: Thomas.

Buchanan, W. W. & Irvine, W. J. (1967). Symposium on auto-immunity and genetics. *Clin. exp. Immun.* **2,** Suppl.

Burnet, F. M. (1959). *The Clonal Selection Theory of Acquired Immunity.* Cambridge University Press.

East, June. (1969). Viruses and auto-immunity. *Vox Sang,* **16,** 318.

Glynn, L. E. & Holborow, E. J. (1964). *Auto-immunity.* Oxford: Blackwell.

Humphrey, J. H. & White, R. G. (1969). *Immunology for Students of Medicine,* p. 600. Oxford: Blackwell.

Irvine, W. J. (1967). Immunobiology of the thymus and its relation to auto-immune disease. In *Modern Trends in Immunology, 2,* p. 250. Ed. Cruickshank, R. & Weir, D. M. London: Butterworth.

Perlmann, P. (1969). Bacteria and auto-immunity. *Vox Sang,* **16,** 314.

Roitt, I. M. (1969). Humoral immunity and auto-immune disease. *Vox Sang,* **16,** 341.

Samter, M. (1965). *Immunologic Diseases.* Boston: Little Brown.

Trentin, J. J. (1967). *Cross-reacting Antigens and Neo-antigens (with Implications for Auto-immunity and Cancer Immunity).* Baltimore: Williams & Wilkins.

Turk, J. L. (1969). *Immunology in Clinical Medicine.* London: Heinemann.

Turk, J. L. (1969). Cellular immunity and auto-immune diseases. *Vox Sang,* **16,** 341.

Weir, D. M. (1969). Altered antigen and auto-immunity. *Vox Sang,* **16,** 304.

Whaley, K. & Dick, W. C. (1969). Rheumatoid arthritis: aetiological and pathogenic considerations. *Br. J. hosp. Med.* **2,** 1916.

Chapter 10

IMMUNOHAEMATOLOGY

Knowledge of blood groups in man and animals has been very closely associated with the development of the science of immunology. Differences between the red blood cells of animals were first noted in goats as early as 1900 when Ehrlich and Morgenroth immunized 'a strong male goat' with nearly a litre of blood obtained from three other goats. The serum which they obtained from the immunized goat lysed the cells of all but one of the nine goats they tested. However, to Ehrlich the most important finding was that the cells of the immunized goat itself were completely unaffected. This proved to him that an animal would not produce autoantibodies against its own tissues and so destroy itself. It was left to Karl Landsteiner who made the same observations in humans to take up the detailed study of these antigenic differences. Landsteiner's important work on the immunochemical determinants of antigenic specificity stems from this period and still stands today as of fundamental value to our understanding of antigens. Studies in blood group serology have led to the development of a large variety of techniques which have wide application to immunological problems outside this field. Notable amongst these is the antiglobulin test devised by Coombs and his associates by means of which enormous advances have been made in many branches of immunology. Study of the development of blood group antibodies in serum has thrown light on the mechanisms underlying the formation of natural antibodies. Apart from these contributions to the understanding of immunological problems, information on blood groups has important implications in genetics and in forensic studies.

117

Blood Groups

ABO antigens and isoantibodies

The ABO blood group system was described as a result of Landsteiner's demonstration of four distinct groups of agglutination reaction between human red blood cells and normal human serum. The differences in agglutination were due to the presence or absence of two antigens A and B on the red cell membrane. The four combinations which result from this are: (1) the presence of A antigen in the absence of B – Group A cells; (2) the presence of B antigen in the absence of A – Group B cells; (3) the presence of both A and B antigens – Group AB cells; and (4) the absence of both A and B antigens – Group O cells.

The sera of individuals also contain natural antibodies able to react with, and agglutinate if present in sufficient concentration, the cells of other individuals of different blood group.

These natural antibodies or isoantibodies are formed shortly after birth and appear to be stimulated by immunization with A and B antigens derived from the normal bacterial flora of the gut. Antigens with blood group specificity are widely distributed in nature (see also p. 16).

From a consideration of the phenomenon of immunological tolerance and the fact that an individual is tolerant to 'self' antigens (Chap. 9) it can be seen that an individual will respond only to an antigen to which he is not already tolerant. Thus an individual with blood group A cells will be tolerant to the A antigen and will therefore respond only to the B antigen derived from the gut flora. The same holds for blood group B individuals who can respond only to the A antigen.   ...

Thus individuals of blood Group A will have isoantibodies of blood group B specificity, i.e. anti-B antibodies, and blood group B individuals will in the same way have anti-A isoantibodies. Blood group O individuals whose immune system will not have developed tolerance to either A or B antigens will have, as would be expected, both anti-A and anti-B isoagglutinins.

The blood group antigens A and B occur not only in the red cells but are widely distributed in the tissues with the exception of the central nervous system. Just under 80 per cent of individuals also have one of these antigens (corresponding to their blood group) in the tissue fluids and secretions (except CSF). Chemical studies on these antigens recovered in quantity from ovarian cyst fluid show them to be glycoproteins and that the difference between A and B substances is determined by the nature of a single saccharide attached to the terminal sugar of the glycoprotein chain. Group O individuals secrete a glycoprotein (H-substance) which is probably the basic chain structure material from which A and B substances are derived by the addition of the specific saccharides (p. 18).

Blood transfusion in relation to ABO groups

Transfusion of an individual with red cells from an individual of a different group results in exposure of the transfused cells to an isoagglutinin – anti-A or anti-B – and except in the case of O cells which carry neither the A nor the B antigen, the cells will be destroyed with resulting haemoglobinaemia and haemo-globinuria. Although it is clearly best to administer blood only of the same group as the recipient, in an emergency Group O cells can be given. Although the plasma of a Group O individual (sometimes called a 'universal donor') contains anti-A and anti-B isoagglutinins, these are so diluted by the recipient's plasma (a pint of blood would be diluted about 1 in 12) to have only a negligible effect except when large quantities of blood have to be administered. Group O individuals whose serum contains anti-A and anti-B isoagglutinins cannot accept blood of any group except O. Since an individual of group AB has neither anti-A nor anti-B isoantibodies he can accept blood of any of the four groups and has therefore been called a 'universal recipient'.

This relatively straightforward scheme is unfortunately slightly complicated by the existence of a number of subgroups of A (probably five in all). However only A_1 and A_2 are of importance as far as transfusion is concerned. The frequency of occurrence in Caucasians of the six different ABO groups is shown below.

BLOOD GROUP	FREQUENCY	Isoantibodies
O	43.5%	Anti-A ($+$Anti-A_1), Anti-B
A_1	34.8%	Anti-B
A_2	9.6%	Anti-B (occasionally Anti-A_1)
B	8.5%	Anti-A ($+$Anti-A_1)
A_1B	2.5%	None
A_2B	0.8%	None (occasionally Anti-A_1)

The Rhesus blood group system

This system is the next most important system to the ABO groups. The Rh blood group antigens are present in the red cells of 85 per cent of Caucasians and 94 per cent of Negroes. The most common of the Rhesus antigens are C, c, D, d, E, e, and the table shows some of the various combinations which can exist and their frequency in Caucasians.

GENOTYPE		FREQUENCY	
CDe / cde	–	31.7%	
CDe / CDe	–	16.6%	Rh-positive
CDe / cDe	–	11.5%	
cDE / cde	–	10.9%	
cde / cde	–	15.1%	Rh-negative

The Rhesus group of an individual must be taken into account for transfusion purposes. Of these antigens D is the most potent although immunization by D and at the same time by the C or E antigens can occur. A variant of D named D^u has been described and cells carrying this antigen are not agglutinated by routine anti-D sera. For transfusion purposes recipients carrying the D^u antigen are considered to be Rh-negative, whilst donors in this category are regarded as Rh-positive.

Rhesus incompatibility

The clinical importance of the Rhesus groups lies in the ability of the red cells of a Rhesus-positive foetus to immunize its Rhesus-negative mother. Immunization usually takes place following the trauma of parturition with the result that the maternal immune response does not develop until a *second* pregnancy. The maternal anti-Rh antibody is passed to the new foetus via the placenta and causes haemolytic destruction of its erythrocytes. This condition is known as haemolytic disease of the newborn or erythroblastosis foetalis. Since the original description of the disease it has been found that blood group antigen systems other than the Rh system can be responsible for the condition. For example a group O mother can occasionally be immunized by foetal antigens if the father is A_1, A_1B or B.

The serious nature of haemolytic disease of the newborn necessitating complete exchange of the infant's blood (exchange transfusion) to remove the maternal antibody, has now been alleviated by a rather ingenious immunological manoeuvre. This is based on the observation that attempted immunization by an antigen in the presence of its specific antibody tends to inhibit synthesis of the antibody to the injected antigen. It is known for example that immunization of infants is best delayed for a few months after birth to allow the levels of maternal antibody to fall.

In the case of a recognized Rhesus incompatibility it is now the practice to give a small dose of potent anti-Rh antibody to immunized Rh-negative mothers within three days after delivery of an Rh-positive infant. The antibody appears to inhibit the response to the Rhesus antigen, possibly by diverting the cells carrying the antigen from the antibody-forming tissues or perhaps by a direct 'feedback inhibition' effect on the antibody-forming cells. This treatment has been very successful in clinical trials and the future outlook is very hopeful so that the disease may soon become of only historical interest.

The detection of anti-Rh antibodies

After the recognition of the association between haemolytic disease of the newborn and Rhesus immunization it soon became apparent that the standard method of demonstrating anti-Rh antibody – by direct agglutination of a saline suspension of Rh-positive cells by serum from an immunized mother – was not able to show up the presence of antibody in one-half to two-thirds of sera tested. A solution to the problem was found by the substitution of a dilute protein solution, e.g. bovine albumen, for the normal saline diluent. Visible agglutination could then be readily demonstrated in the majority of cases. The form of serum antibody responsible for agglutination demonstrable only in protein diluent, became known as 'incomplete' antibody in contrast to the saline-active 'complete' antibody. The incomplete antibody was thought of initially as univalent, having only one antibody-binding site, but it has now been shown to be IgG antibody of normal bivalent structure (p. 43); the complete anti-red cell antibody on the other hand has been shown to be IgM in nature. It seems that the smaller molecular weight IgG antibody is not readily able to link together red cells in suspension unless the mutually repellent effect of red cells, which normally keeps them in suspension in a saline medium, is reduced by altering their surface charge by the addition of protein. In contrast the much larger, multivalent IgM antibodies have a considerably greater chance of bringing about agglutination.

Another very important method for demonstrating incomplete antibodies is the Coombs antiglobulin test. An antiserum is prepared in rabbits against human immunoglobulins and this is used to react with Rh-positive cells, coated with human incomplete antibody, bringing about their agglutination simply by linking together the molecules of human globulin still attached to the red cells (p. 141 and Fig. 30).

One of the advantages of this method is that it can be used to detect the coating *in vivo* of Rh-positive cells by small amounts of antibody. After the cells have been thoroughly washed they are mixed with the anti-human globulin serum which will bring about agglutination of cells with human globulin attached to their surface. This form of the test is known as the 'direct Coombs test'. Another form of the test is used to detect incomplete anti-Rh antibodies in the serum of a patient who has been immunized against Rh antigens. Rh-positive cells are simply mixed with the patient's serum and if anti-Rh antibody is present the cells will be agglutinated by the subsequent addition of an anti-human globulin serum. This variation is known as the 'indirect Coombs test'.

Other blood group systems

In 1927 Landsteiner described two human antigens M and N. The use of antisera against these antigens can divide individuals into three types, half of whom have the MN genotype and 28 per cent and 22 per cent respectively have MM and NN genotypes. A further antigen was later found, the S antigen, and the group is known as the MNS blood group system. This group is of limited clinical importance although a few instances of haemolytic disease of the newborn have been reported due to incompatibility of these antigens.

Landsteiner's P antigen is noteworthy because a naturally occurring anti-P cold agglutinin is found in a large proportion of the 20 per cent of individuals who are P-negative. Amongst a number of blood group systems described including those of

Lutheran, Kell, Lewis, Kidd, Duffy and Diego, special mention should be made of the Lewis system because naturally occurring antibodies to Lewis antigens are frequently found in human serum. They sometimes act as cold agglutinins and have been found occasionally to be the cause of haemolytic transfusion reactions. These antigens are unique in that they are not part of the red cell structure but are soluble antigens found in body fluids, which adsorb on to the red cell surface.

Antigens of blood leucocytes and platelets

As has been discussed in the section on transplantation antigens, blood leucocytes in man carry the major histocompatibility antigen system HL-A. The appearance of antibodies against donor leucocytes and also platelet antigens is a common finding after blood transfusion. This results in rapid destruction of the transfused cells and although immunization occurs more frequently than anti-red cell immunization the consequences are less dangerous.

Leucocyte and platelet groups fall into two types: those which they share in common with red cells, and those which are restricted to leucocytes and platelets and other tissue cells. The blood group antigens A and B are the main antigens shared with erythrocytes. The important antigenic group limited to leucocytes, platelets and other tissue cells is the HL-A system.

A reaction between anti-leucocyte isoantibodies and transfused leucocytes often gives rise to febrile transfusion reactions and their incidence can be correlated with the number of transfusions given. Although these reactions are not usually severe they can be a disadvantage to patients for whom repeated transfusions are necessary. In this situation the simplest solution is to remove the majority of leucocytes from the blood by separation of red cells which can be readily sedimented by the addition of gelatin. This is preferable to the complex serological procedures required to assure compatibility of leucocytes.

The transfusion of fresh platelets is of value in patients suffering from haemorrhagic disorders due to thrombocytopoenia, and although, theoretically, selection of compatible platelets is desirable, in practice platelets are usually obtained from a small number of donors, if possible related to the recipient.

123

The HL-A system of antigens is of considerable current interest to immunologists because of their importance as histo-compatibility antigens. Unfortunately the HL-A system appears to be the most complex system of this type ever known to man. It is the equivalent of the H-2 system in the mouse (p. 83) and of the other main histocompatibility systems known to exist in other mammalian species.

Between 15 and 20 more or less well-defined antigens have been identified in the HL-A system, and more than 100 pheno-types have been found within this system. Despite these com-plexities as more experience is gained in the grouping procedures (leucoagglutination by a panel of antisera), and supplies of suitable antisera become more widely available, it seems likely that by accumulating a list of available fully typed donors, and with improvements in storage and preservation of tissues it may eventually become possible to select from amongst the many possible variations a suitable donor for each recipient.

FURTHER READING

Dausset, J. & Colombani, J. (1967). White cells and platelets in transfusion immunology. In *Modern Trends in Immunology, 2*, p. 314. Ed. Cruick-shank, R. & Weir, D. M. London: Butterworth.

Race, R. R. & Sanger, R. (1968). *Blood Groups in Man,* 5th ed. Oxford: Blackwell.

WHO (1967). The suppression of Rh-immunization by passively administered human immunoglobulin (IgG) anti-D (anti-Rh_0). *Bull. Wld Hlth Org.* **36,** 467.

Chapter 11

MALIGNANT DISEASE

In discussing the general biological significance of immune reactions in maintaining the integrity of the cellular systems of the body, Burnet points out that in man, in whom more than 10^{14} cells are constantly reproducing, there is sufficient evidence to make it likely that at any given genetic locus an error occurs with a frequency in the range of 10^{-5} to 10^{-7} per replication. This means that in the cell population there must be many millions of errors or mutations occurring every day of life. It seems inconceivable that complex and long-lived multicellular animals could have evolved unless some means of dealing with this eventually had been developed.

The role of immunological mechanisms in the suppression of malignant cells has been appreciated since the work of Paul Ehrlich at the beginning of the century, but it is only in the last ten years or so that immunologists have begun to unravel the details of the immunological processes underlying the control of tumours, the antigenic changes in tumour cells themselves, and the extent and activities of the immune response arising as a result of these changes.

Evidence for the role of immune mechanisms

Mention is made in Chapter 8 of the increased incidence in thymectomized mice of tumours induced by chemical carcinogens and viruses. This seems likely to be due to a deficiency of the cell-mediated immune mechanisms which lie under the control of the thymus (p. 56). These neonatally thymectomized animals are unable to reject incompatible tissue grafts and do not give delayed hypersensitivity reactions of the tuberculin type. These activities depend on intact cell-mediated, thymus-dependent immune reactivity and it is the absence of this reactivity which allows tumour cells to grow unhindered.

Another example where deficiency of the cell-mediated immune mechanisms is associated with tumour formation is in a condition known as graft-versus-host disease. This condition is produced in mice by injecting spleen cells into an unrelated recipient, the reaction of the spleen cells against the host resulting in destruction of its lymphoid tissues. This can be demonstrated by using two inbred strains of mice, e.g. CBA and C57 Black, and injecting the spleen cells of one of the parents into the offspring of such a mating. CBA cells injected into a CBA/C57B recipient will recognize the C57B component of the post-lymphoid cells as foreign but will not be themselves rejected because the recipient itself carries the CBA antigens.

The destruction of the recipient's lymphoid tissues and thus its cell-mediated immune response, produces a defect in the control of neoplastic cell proliferation and the mice frequently develop tumours of the lymphoid tissues having many of the features of Hodgkin's disease of the human.

A similar atrophy of the lymphoid tissues has been described in mice infected with reoviruses and the animals have an increased incidence of tumours compared with non-infected strains of mice. A reovirus (Epstein Barr) has been isolated from the human lymphoid tumour known as Burkitt's lymphoma and it has been proposed that the tumour is of virus origin induced perhaps in the way described above. Recent evidence in patients with Burkitt's lymphoma has added considerable support to the significance of cell-mediated immune mechanisms in the control of the tumour. Only one of twelve patients on skin testing with extracts of their own cells gave positive delayed hypersensitivity reactions. However when the tumour growth was suppressed with cyclophosphamide, skin tests became positive in seven of the twelve indicating a recovery of the cell-mediated immune mechanisms which is associated with remission of the tumour.

There is as yet no firm evidence that tumours in humans are caused by viruses; however recent work in America suggests the possible role of a virus as a cause of mammary carcinoma. Virus particles with similar morphology have been identified in occasional specimens of normal human and mouse milk, and women with a family history of mammary carcinoma have a markedly increased incidence of the virus in their milk. The role of immune mechanisms in controlling the tumour is suggested by tests in which sera from normal men, and women with breast cancer, were incubated with mouse mammary tumour virus. Tumour-inducing activity of the virus in mice was found to be reduced in the samples treated with the sera from women with tumours.

A somewhat disturbing result of the use of anti-lymphocytic serum (ALS) in man for immunosuppression in tissue transplantation (p. 88), is the small but significantly increased incidence of tumours in such individuals and it seems probable that this is due to suppression of immunological surveillance mechanisms. It is also interesting to note that various chemical immunosuppressive drugs and X-rays, acting like ALS on the lymphoid tissues, are in many instances carcinogens as well as immunosuppressive agents.

The incidence of cancer in man is highest at the two extremes of life and it is just at these times that the immune system is least efficient. All these observations point to the probable important role played by the intact immune mechanisms in maintaining the body free of undesirable mutant neoplastic cells.

Tumour antigens

It can be deduced from the foregoing discussion that for the immunological system to react against tumour cells, these cells must be changed in some way so that they are no longer recognized as self. That this is indeed so is substantiated by many examples of tumours which have been found to develop new antigens as part of their cell structure. There are two types of antigenic change: (1) where the specificity of the new antigen is dependent on the inducing agent such as a virus, and (2) tumours induced by chemical carcinogens in which the antigenic change induced by the same carcinogen in two different animals is different in each case.

There are numerous examples of tumour formation which seem to be associated with these changes. The SV_{40} virus induces tumours in monkeys, the Rous sarcoma virus in chickens and the polyoma virus in mice. The tumours induced in mice by the polyoma virus have recently been shown to consist of two sorts of cells – cells that are malignant on introduction into another mouse and cells that do not survive transplantation. It seems possible that the latter cells are destroyed by the immune system because they carry recognizable foreign antigens on their surface.

When cells of the non-transplantable variety are cultured *in vitro* variants appear which have lost their antigenicity and can thus transfer the tumour. This raises the possibility that attempts to eliminate malignant cells by increasing the immune reaction against them may result in the 'selection' of 'non-antigenic' variants which would allow the tumour to spread.

The tumour-specific antigens are comparable to the weak histocompatibility antigens (p. 83) and their strength has been found to vary for different aetiological groups. Methylcholanthrene-induced sarcomas in mice have been found to be more strongly antigenic than similar sarcomas induced by dibenzanthracene. Among the virus tumours, Moloney virus-induced lymphomas of the mouse are quite strongly antigenic whereas the Gross agent induces a similar tumour with very weak tumour specific antigens. Consistent with the finding that the specificity of tumour antigens varies even with one chemical carcinogen is the finding that the strength of these antigens varies also.

Having established that antigenic changes occur in neoplastic cells and that immunological processes are apparently involved in the body's reaction to tumours, the question is how in fact does any tumour grow and spread throughout the body in the face of the body's immune reaction? Some of the factors which tip the balance in favour of tumour growth have already been discussed in relation to central defects of the immune response.

Another important factor is that the tumour-specific antigens are often not strongly antigenic and the degree of immunity developed is insufficient to cause the rejection of a rapidly growing tumour. In experiments in mice, with primary tumours induced by chemical carcinogens, it has been shown that if a mouse is pre-immunized with tumour cells (inactivated by X-irradiation) the animal can then develop a state of immunity to transfer of living tumour cells provided that the number of transferred cells is not too large to overcome the induced immunity.

Implications in cancer therapy

The classical treatment for carcinoma of the breast and many other tumours is the radical surgical removal of the neoplastic tissue and much of the surrounding tissue, including the lymph glands of the area.

It is now recognized that this treatment sometimes enhances the spread of secondary deposits, and it is thought that this might be due to removal of lymphoid tissues involved in the immune response to the antigens of the tumour, and possibly also to diminution in the antigenic stimulus to the immune system. The balance is thus tipped in favour of remaining tumour cells which can proliferate unchecked. In addition it should be remembered that mammary carcinogenesis almost certainly also involves the interplay of a variety of non-immunological factors – hormonal, genetic and possibly viral as suggested above.

A number of ways have been proposed of inhibiting tumour growth by enhancing the immune response to the tumour antigens either by active immunization with tumour antigens or by non-specifically stimulating the lymphoid tissues. This area is fraught with ethical and practical difficulties but a few partially successful, albeit heroic, experiments have been tried in man.

In one small series in America, malignant tissue was interchanged between pairs of patients with 'incurable' tumours. After allowing sufficient time for an immune response, leucocytes from the immunized individual were injected into the original donor of the tumour tissue. Clinical benefit was claimed in 5 of the 14 patients involved, one patient having complete remission with the disappearance of the numerous secondary tumour deposits of a malignant melanoma with no sign of a recurrence after one year. The spontaneous disappearance of tumours and complete recovery of patients with widespread cancer does on rare occasions happen and is usually explained as divine intervention. A more readily acceptable explanation of such phenomena is that for some reason the balance between tumour growth and the immune reaction against it has been tipped in favour of the immune response. It is also necessary to judge the result of experiments such as those cited above with this possibility in mind.

FURTHER READING

Alexander, P. & Hamilton Fairley, G. (1968). The allergic response in malignant disease. In *Clinical aspects of Immunology*, 2nd ed. Ed. Gell, P. G. H. & Coombs, R. R. A. Oxford: Blackwell.

Burnet, Sir Macfarlane (1962). *The Integrity of the Body*. London: Oxford University Press.

Burnet, Sir Macfarlane (1970). *Immunological Surveillance*. London: Pergamon Press.

Fenner, F. (1968). *The Pathogenesis and Ecology of Viral Infection*. New York: Academic Press.

Trentin, J. J. (1967). *Cross-reacting Antigens and Neo-antigens (with Implications for Auto-immunity and Cancer Immunity)*. Baltimore: Williams & Wilkins.

Turk, J. L. (1969). *Immunology in Clinical Medicine*. London: Heinemann.

Chapter 12

THE INTERACTION OF ANTIBODY WITH ANTIGEN

An antibody, as has been pointed out, is an immunoglobulin molecule secreted into the tissue fluids from lymphoid cells which have been exposed to a foreign substance – an antigen. An antigen may be potentially harmful, such as a bacterium or virus, or it may be a harmless bland substance such as foreign serum protein. The antibody can combine only with antigen which is identical or nearly identical with the inducing antigen and not with unrelated antigens. When molecules of antibody and antigen are brought together in solution, they interact with each other by the formation of a link between an antigen-binding site on the immunoglobulin molecule – part of the Fab fragment – and the particular chemical groupings which make up what is termed the antigenic determinant of the antigen molecule. The molecules are held together by non-covalent intermolecular forces which are effective only when the antigen-binding site and the antigenic determinant group are able to make close contact. The better the fit the closer the contact and the stronger the antigen-antibody bond, these factors determining what is often called the affinity of the antibody molecule; antibodies of varying combining quality exist and the overall tendency to combine with antigen is the average ability of the antibodies to combine with antigen or the average intrinsic association constant. This can be calculated experimentally by application of the concepts of chemical equilibria to antigen-antibody interactions. Studies of this type have shown that the affinity of antibodies increases as immunization proceeds and that the dose of antigen can influence the quality of antibody.

The methods used for the detection of antigen-antibody reactions in the laboratory fall into two functional groups: first, procedures designed to elucidate the cytodynamics of antibody formation which involve the study of the behaviour of single cells or small populations of cells; the second group, which is the subject of the present discussion, concerns the detection and quantitation of *secreted antibody* circulating in the blood or present in the tissue fluids.

The methods used here range in their application from highly specialized studies of the physico-chemical aspects of antigen-antibody interaction to widely used procedures designed to aid in the diagnosis of disease.

Primary interaction and secondary effects

In practical terms, the union of antibody with antigen can be detected at two different levels. The first level is that following *primary union* of the two reactants and usually requires that one or other reactant is labelled with a suitable marker such as a fluorescent dye or a radioactive isotope. A simple example of this is the microscopic localization in a tissue of a particular micro-organism utilizing an antiserum prepared against the micro-organism and labelled with a dye that fluoresces under UV light.

The second level at which antigen-antibody combination can be detected depends on the development, after primary union, of certain changes in the physical state of the complex, resulting in precipitation or agglutination of the components or, alternatively, in the activation of non-antibody components such as serum complement or histamine from mast cells. Reactions of this type occurring subsequent to primary union are termed *secondary phenomena*. This discussion is concerned with the principles of a few of these secondary phenomena which are in common use.

Secondary effects; interpretation and applications

Before considering these reactions individually, it is important to be aware of the difficulties in interpreting results of such tests. The initiation and development of the secondary phenomena constitute a complicated series of events involving many variables such as the type of antibody taking part, the relative proportions of antibody and antigen, characteristics of the antigen molecule, presence of electrolytes, inhibitory substances and unstable components.

Despite these formidable difficulties, the widely and long used secondary phenomena such as precipitation, agglutination and complement fixation have an important role to play as aids in the diagnosis of disease and in the identification of microorganisms.

The secondary phenomena, as already indicated, can bring about several readily observable changes when carried out *in vitro* and these are used in tests to demonstrate the presence of antibody in the sera of patients suffering from infectious disease, or producing an antibody response to cell antigens as might, for example, occur after incompatible blood transfusion, tissue grafting or in autoimmune states.

Reactions of this type can also be used to identify antigens in the tissues or body fluids and, for example, would be utilized for blood grouping, tissue typing or the identification of microorganisms.

Among the most important of these reactions are *precipitation*, which occurs between antibody and antigen molecules in soluble form; *agglutination*, in which the antibodies directed against surface antigens of particulate materials such as microorganisms or erythrocytes, link them together in large clumps or aggregates; and *complement fixation* in which antibody molecules, after reaction with antigen, activate the complex blood components which make up serum complement.

In addition to these widely used serological tests, a number of other effects of antigen-antibody interaction are of medical importance. These include neutralization tests used for example in virus identification, immobilization tests with bacteria and protozoa and skin tests for the reaginic antibody characteristic of anaphylactic states.

Precipitation

Optimal proportions

As a result of the interaction of antibody and antigen molecules in solution, complexes of the two types of molecule will form and precipitation may occur depending on the relative concentration of the two reactants. If a series of tubes is set up (Fig. 23), each containing a constant amount of antiserum, and decreasing amounts of antigen are added to the tubes in the row, a haziness will start to appear in the tubes gradually increasing to clearly visible aggregates or precipitates. The amount of precipitation will be seen to increase along the row, reaching a

Antibody Neat in each tube.

Fig. 23

maximum and then falling off with the lower antigen concentration. The tubes where most precipitate appears contain the *optimal proportions* of antigen and antibody for precipitation and the proportions are constant for all dilutions of the same reagents. The composition of the precipitate varies with the original proportions of the antibody and antigen; if antigen is in excess the precipitate will contain relatively more of this component and similarly more antibody if it is present in excess. As can be seen from Figure 24, on the antigen excess side of optimal proportions less precipitate appears and this is due to the inability of the antigen-antibody complexes formed to link up to other complexes and so make a large aggregate or lattice which will appear as a visible precipitate (tube 1 Fig. 24). Large aggregates of antibody and antigen can form best under conditions of optimal proportions where the antibody and antigen proportions are such that after initial combination of the molecules, free antigen-binding sites and antigen determinant groups remain, enabling the complexes to link up into a large lattice formation (as in tube 2 of Fig. 24). In antibody excess all the free determinants of the antigen molecule are soon taken up with antibody, so that very little linking can take place between the complexes (as in tube 3 of Fig. 24).

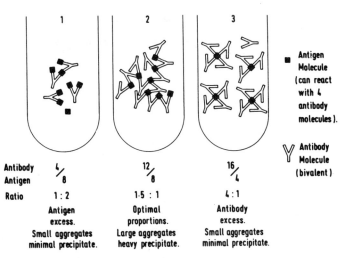

	1	**2**	**3**
Antibody	4	12	16
Antigen	8	8	4
Ratio	1 : 2	1·5 : 1	4 : 1
	Antigen excess.	Optimal proportions.	Antibody excess.
	Small aggregates minimal precipitate.	Large aggregates heavy precipitate.	Small aggregates minimal precipitate.

■ Antigen Molecule (can react with 4 antibody molecules).

Y Antibody Molecule (bivalent)

Fig. 24

Applications

The precipitin test can be carried out in a quantitative manner by estimating the protein content of the precipitate at optimal proportions. The qualitative test is much more widely used and is of considerable value in detecting and identifying antigens, having applications in the typing of streptococci or pneumococci. This is done by layering an extract of the organism over anti-serum. After a short while, a ring of precipitate forms at the interface (this is called the ring test). The technique is also used in forensic studies and in detecting adulteration of foodstuffs. A modification of the test in which precipitation is allowed to occur in *agar gel* is very widely used for detecting the presence of antibody in serum or antigen in unknown preparations, and is valuable for showing the identity of different antigen preparations (Fig. 25). A concentration gradient forms in the gel, the concentration of a substance decreasing as the molecules diffuse away from the well in which they were placed. Precipitin bands form in the gel in the position where the antigen and antibody molecules reach optimal proportions after diffusion. When a large number of different antigens are present in a solution, it is difficult to separate the precipitin bands for each of the antigen-antibody reactions by the simple gel-diffusion method just

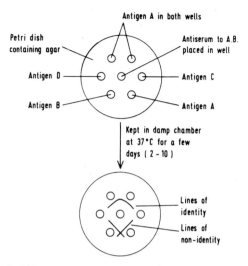

Precipitin bands form where antigen and antibody reach optimal proportions after diffusion towards each other. No reaction occurs with unrelated antigens C and D.

Fig. 25 Immunodiffusion or gel diffusion test. Wells are cut in a layer of agar in a Petri dish. Antiserum and antigen solutions are placed opposite each other in the wells and after allowing a few days for diffusion to take place precipitin bands will form where antibody and antigen meet in suitable proportions (optimal proportions). No reactions take place with antigens C and D as the antiserum in the central well contains antibodies only for antigens A and B. Lines of identity as formed between the two A wells enable the technique to be used for identifying unknown antigens.

described. In such a situation, a variation of this method can be used to identify the individual components. This modification is particularly valuable in analysing a multicomponent system such as serum. The individual components of serum are first separated by electrophoresis in agar gel and an antiserum, prepared against the serum, is allowed to diffuse towards the separated components, resulting in the formation of precipitin bands (Fig. 26). This method, known as immunoelectrophoresis, is particularly valuable for showing the presence of abnormal globulin constituents in the serum of patients with myelomatosis and other serum protein abnormalities.

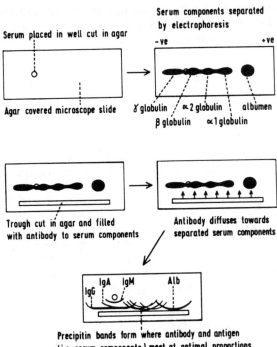

Serum placed in well cut in agar

Serum components separated by electrophoresis

−ve   +ve

Agar covered microscope slide

ɣ globulin   ∝2 globulin   albumen
β globulin   ∝1 globulin

Trough cut in agar and filled with antibody to serum components

Antibody diffuses towards separated serum components

IgG IgA IgM   Alb

Precipitin bands form where antibody and antigen (i.e. serum components) meet at optimal proportions. Approximately 30 components can be detected in human serum in this way. The position of the main immunoglobulins is shown.

Fig. 26 Immunoelectrophoresis. The antigen, for example, serum, is placed in a small well cut in a layer of agar on a microscope slide. A direct current is applied and differential migration of the serum components takes place. (They are not normally visible in the agar and will show up only if suitably stained.) After electrophoresis for an hour or so, a trough is cut longitudinally in the agar and an antiserum against the electrophoresed antigen is placed in the trough. The two components diffuse towards each other and precipitin bands form. These can be shown up more clearly by staining with a protein stain. This is a very powerful analytic technique and can show up about 30 different components in human serum compared with 4 or 5 by electrophoresis.

A microimmunodiffusion test with wells cut in a layer of agar on a microscope slide is a convenient modification of the Petri dish method. This procedure has come into wide use for the detection in human serum of the *Australia antigen* which is associated with serum hepatitis. The routine screening of blood products by this technique using specific antisera prepared in animals is likely to become an important laboratory test in the prevention of serum hepatitis outbreaks.

Agglutination

In this reaction the antigen is part of the surface of some particulate material such as a red cell, bacterium or perhaps an inorganic particle (e.g. polystyrene latex) which has been coated with antigen. Antibody added to a suspension of such particles combines with the surface antigens and links them together to form clearly-visible aggregates or agglutinates (Fig. 27). In its simplest form an agglutination test is set up in round-bottomed test tubes or perspex plates with round-bottomed wells and doubling dilutions of the antiserum are made up in the tubes (neat, 1:2, 1:4, 1:8, etc). The particulate antigen is then added

Red blood cells

IgM anti red cell antibody

+

Agglutination

IgM antibody is efficient in bringing about agglutination as it has 5 combining sites.

Red cells   +   Anti red cell antibody   →   Agglutinated red cells

Fig. 27 Agglutination reaction. The IgM molecule with at least five antigen-binding sites is particularly effective in bringing about agglutination.

138

and after incubation at 37°C. agglutination is seen in the bottom of the tubes. The last tube showing clearly visible agglutination is the end point of the test. The reciprocal dilution of the anti-serum at the end point, e.g. 1/256 is known as the *titre* of the antiserum and is a measure of the number of antibody units per unit volume of serum, e.g. if the end point occurs at a 1/256 dilution of the antiserum and if the test has been carried out in 1 ml volumes, the titre of the serum is 256 units per ml of serum. One practical difficulty of importance in agglutination tests is the occasional inhibition of agglutination in the first tubes of an antiserum dilution series, agglutination occurring only in those tubes containing more dilute antiserum. This is known as the *prozone phenomenon* and is probably, in part, due to the stabiliz-ing effects of high protein concentration on the particles, the protein coating the particles, increasing their net charge and so bringing about increased electrostatic repulsion between individual particles, thus opposing the efforts of the antibody molecules to link the particles together. However, once the protein concentration is reduced by dilution the antibody molecules can then exert their aggregating effect and bring about agglutination. The agglutination reaction has been shown to require the presence of electrolytes in the suspending medium and is usually performed for this reason at physiological salt concentration.

Applications

One of the classical applications of the agglutination test in diagnostic bacteriology is the Widal test used for the demon-stration of antibodies to salmonellae in serum specimens taken from suspected enteric fever cases. Agglutination is the basic technique used in blood grouping, the A, B or O group of the red cells under test being determined by agglutination with a specific antiserum – an anti-A serum for example will agglutinate A cells but not B or O cells. Red cells and inert particles such as polystyrene latex can be coated with various antigens and suit-ably coated particles are used in a variety of diagnostic tests such as thyroid antibody tests using thyroglobulin-coated cells or latex particles. Hormone-coated red cells or inert particles are used in many hormone assay procedures which are based on the inhibition of the antibody-induced agglutination of the hormone-

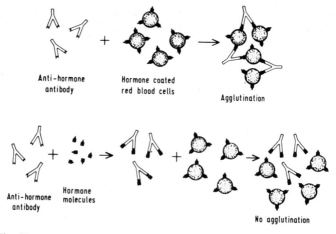

Fig. 28 Principle of hormone assay by agglutination inhibition. Red cells coated with hormone are agglutinable by anti-hormone antibody. The addition to the antiserum of a test sample containing free hormone will block the antigen-binding sites and prevent agglutination. The test can be carried out quantitatively by comparing the activity of a known standard hormone preparation with the test sample.

coated particles by hormone added in the sample under test (Fig. 28). Tests of this type are in wide use in pregnancy diagnosis.

Certain viruses, e.g. the myxoviruses causing influenza and mumps, have the property of bringing about agglutination of red cells (haemagglutination). Inhibition of haemagglutination by antibody in patients' serum is a widely-used diagnostic procedure. The presence of antibody in the patient's serum is thus detected by its ability to link with virus particles and prevent them from bringing about agglutination of the red cells (Fig. 29).

IgM antibodies capable of agglutinating human red cells (including those of the individual producing the antibody) between 0 and 4°C. are sometimes found in certain human diseases including primary atypical pneumonia, malaria, trypanosomiasis and acquired haemolytic anaemia.

The presence of antibody globulin on a red cell may not result in direct agglutination of the cells, for example in some Rh-negative mothers with Rh-positive infants or in acquired

140

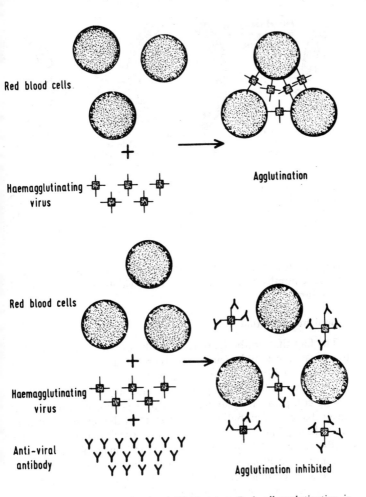

Red blood cells

Haemagglutinating virus

Agglutination

Red blood cells

Haemagglutinating virus

+

Anti-viral antibody

Agglutination inhibited

Fig. 29 Virus haemagglutination inhibition test. Red cell agglutination is brought about by a variety of viruses (see text). This can be inhibited by mixing the virus with anti-viral antibody as shown in the diagram. The test can be quantitated by comparison of serial dilutions of virus alone and virus-antibody mixture.

haemolytic anaemia. It is, however, possible to show that the red cells are coated with antibody by using an antiglobulin serum (produced in the rabbit by injecting human globulin) which will

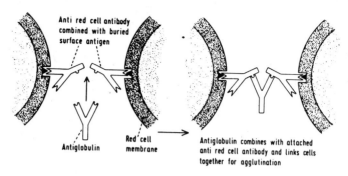

Fig. 30 Coombs antiglobulin test. The red cell antibody, probably because it is directed against an antigen situated deep in the cell wall, cannot link two red cells together for agglutination. The addition of an antiglobulin serum brings about agglutination by linking two attached immunoglobulins to one another.

bring about agglutination of the cells (Fig. 30). This is the basis of the Coombs test which is a very widely used serological procedure.

Complement fixation

The fact that antibody, once it combines with antigen, is able to activate the complement system is used as a way of showing the presence of a particular antibody in a serum, e.g. the Wassermann antibody in syphilis, or in identifying an antigen such as a virus.

The complement system consists of a group of at least nine serum factors of globulin nature present in the serum of normal individuals. The complement of most species will react with antibody derived from other species and guinea-pig serum is a common laboratory source of complement – some of the components of complement are heat labile and are destroyed by heating at 56°C. for 20–30 minutes. The individual components of the complement system are taken up by the antigen-antibody complex in a particular order and destruction of the heat-labile components which are taken up early prevents the remaining components from taking part (see p. 12).

For most antigens the reaction of the complement system with the antigen-antibody complex causes in itself no visible effect, and it is necessary to use an indicator system consisting of sheep red cells coated with anti-sheep red cell antibody. Complement has the ability to lyse the antibody-coated cells, probably by virtue of the esterase activity of one of the components acting on the red cell membrane. In a test the antibody, complement and antigen are first mixed together and after a period of incubation the indicator system, antibody-coated sheep cells, are added. The complement will, however, have been taken up during the incubation stage by the original antibody-antigen complex and will not be available to lyse the red cells. Thus, a positive complement fixation test is indicated by absence of lysis of the red cells whilst a negative test, with unused complement, is shown by lysis of the red cells (Fig. 31).

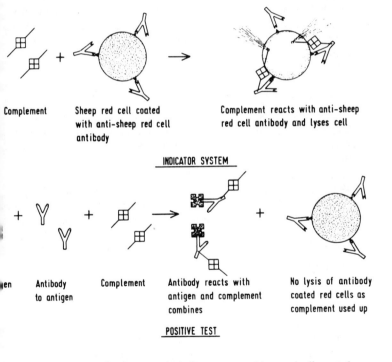

Complement   Sheep red cell coated with anti-sheep red cell antibody   Complement reacts with anti-sheep red cell antibody and lyses cell

INDICATOR SYSTEM

+ Antigen + Antibody to antigen + Complement → Antibody reacts with antigen and complement combines + No lysis of antibody coated red cells as complement used up

POSITIVE TEST

Fig. 31 Complement-fixation test. The indicator system (sheep red cells coated with antibody to sheep red cells) is normally lysed in the presence of complement (fresh guinea-pig serum) – top. If another antibody-antigen system is first mixed with the complement it will no longer be available to lyse the indicator system – bottom.

143

The classical complement fixation test is the Wassermann reaction used in the diagnosis of syphilis in which the test system consists of Wassermann antigen mixed with dilutions of the patient's serum in the presence of guinea-pig complement. After the antigen and patient's serum have had time to react and take up the limited amount of complement available in the system, the indicator system is added to show whether or not there is free complement. Controls are included to ensure that none of the reagents are anti-complementary (able to take up complement non-specifically as might, for example, occur with contaminated serum) and positive and negative control sera are tested in parallel. Complement fixation tests are used routinely for detecting viruses in tissue cultures which have been inoculated with specimens of blood or tissue fluids from humans with probable virus infections.

Antigen-antibody reactions using fluorescent labels

The precise localization of tissue antigens or the antigens of infecting organisms in the body, of anti-tissue antibody and of antigen-antibody complexes was achieved by the introduction of the use of fluorochrome-labelled proteins by Coons and Kaplan in 1950. The adsorption of ultra-violet light between 290 and 495 mμ by fluorescein and its emission of longer wavelength green light (525 mμ) is used to visualize protein labelled with this dye. The technique is more sensitive than precipitation or complement fixation techniques, and fluorescent protein tracers can be detected at a concentration of the order of 1 μg protein per ml body fluid.

Applications

Some of the uses to which the technique has been put include the localization of the origin of a variety of serum protein components, for example immunoglobulin production by plasma cells and other lymphoid cells. The demonstration and localization in the tissues of antibody globulin in a variety of auto-immune conditions has been shown, including an anti-nuclear antibody in the serum of patients with systemic lupus erythematosus and thyroid auto-antibodies in the sera of patients with Hashimoto's thyroiditis. In the diagnostic field most human pathogens can be demonstrated by immunofluorescence and a tentative diagnosis may be made much sooner than by cultivation; the fluorescent method at present can be used to supplement rather than replace conventional methods.

There are two main procedures in use, the direct and indirect methods (Fig. 32). The *direct method* consists of bringing

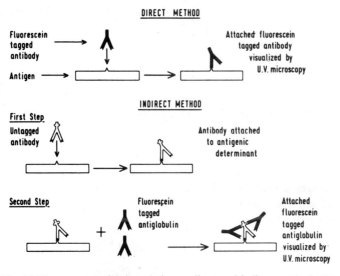

Fig. 32 Fluorescent antibody technique – direct and indirect methods. The indirect method can be seen to be more sensitive as two or more fluorescein-tagged antiglobulin molecules can be attached to each immunoglobulin molecule bound to its antigen.

fluorescein-tagged antibodies into contact with antigens fixed on a slide (e.g. in the form of a tissue section or a smear of an organism), allowing them to react, washing off excess antibody and examining under the UV light microscope. The site of union of the labelled antibody with its antigen can be seen by the apple-green fluorescent areas on the slide. The *indirect method* can be used both for detecting specific antibodies in sera or other body fluids and also for identifying antigens. This method differs

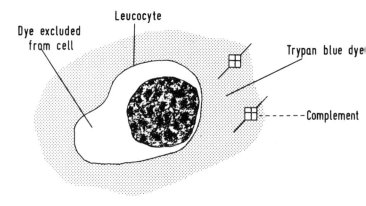

Dye excluded from cell

Leucocyte

Trypan blue dye

Complement

NEGATIVE TEST - No antibody

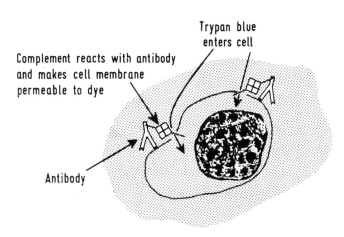

Trypan blue enters cell

Complement reacts with antibody and makes cell membrane permeable to dye

Antibody

POSITIVE TEST - Antibody present

Fig. 33 Cytotoxic test.

from the direct method in the use of a non-labelled antiserum which is layered on first, in the same way as described above. Whether or not this antiserum has reacted with the material on the slide is shown by means of a fluorescein-tagged *antiglobulin serum* specific for the globulin of the serum applied first. Such an antiglobulin serum can be used to detect antibody globulin in sera to a variety of different antigens which gives it a considerable advantage over the direct test; it is also more sensitive.

Cytotoxic tests

Tests of this type are used in combination with red blood cell agglutination for studying histocompatibility antigen systems in tissue typing.

The cytotoxic test consists essentially of determining whether or not the permeability of cells changes after their incubation with antibody and complement (Fig. 33). Cytotoxic antibody after combination with the target cell will activate complement components and bring about changes in permeability of the cell membrane. The permeability changes can affect the ability of the cell to exclude a dye such as trypan blue which will penetrate the cell and be visible by simple microscopic examination.

Although the test is applicable to a wide range of nucleated cells and is the test of choice with blood leucocytes, it is rather less sensitive than the red cell haemagglutination test and more laborious to perform.

Some Common Diagnostic Applications of Antigen-Antibody Reactions in Medical Microbiology

Agglutination tests

The agglutination test already referred to for the sero-diagnosis of salmonella infections is known as the Widal test. It is usual to test dilutions of the patient's serum against standard suspensions of somatic (O) antigen and flagellar (H) antigen of each organism likely to be encountered in the patient's environment. The test usually becomes positive with both suspensions, a week after the onset of the illness but may be weakly positive with one of the antigens even earlier. The titre in an acute infection rises to a maximum by the end of the third week. Complications in interpretation of the results may arise in patients who have been immunized with typhoid-paratyphoid vaccine (TAB). A rising titre may be of some help in diagnosing an infection; furthermore, some months after immunization the titre of O agglutinins tends to fall off leaving only H agglutinins. Normal sera sometimes have low titres of agglutinins for salmonella organisms and this varies in populations in different parts of the world. These difficulties make the test of questionable diagnostic value and its use is now limited.

Another widely used agglutination test is the Paul-Bunnell reaction. This is used for the diagnosis of infectious mononucleosis in which agglutinins develop for sheep erythrocytes. Normal serum may agglutinate sheep cells in low dilutions and a titre of 128 is taken as suggestive and 256 as positive for the test. In some individuals who have received horse serum as a therapeutic agent (e.g. antitetanus serum) agglutinins develop for sheep cells because of the presence in the horse serum of an antigen very widespread in nature, known as the Forssman antigen. This antigen is present in the red cells of sheep and the cells of a number of other species, including the guinea-pig. The usual way of differentiating the two types of antibody is to mix the serum with minced guinea-pig tissue (usually kidney). This treatment will absorb out the anti-Forssman antibody leaving the anti-sheep cell antibody unaffected. Ox red cells which contain both the Forssman antigen and an antigen similar to that on sheep cells, which reacts with the Paul-Bunnell antibody, will absorb out both types of antibody.

An agglutination test is widely used for the diagnosis of rheumatoid arthritis; the sera of 70–80 per cent of patients with this disease contain an IgM antibody which is able to combine with the IgG globulin from various species. Detection of the antibody depends on the agglutination of sheep red cells or inert particles (polystyrene latex) coated with IgG globulin. Sheep red cells for example may be coated with specific rabbit antibody and will then be agglutinated by the IgM antibody in the rheumatoid patient's serum. The antibody is known as rheumatoid factor. Occasional low titres (less than 16 are found in normal sera, 2–5 per cent) and the test is not entirely specific for rheumatoid arthritis.

Complement fixation tests

These tests, described on page 142 have wide application in the diagnosis of bacterial and viral infections. One of the most commonly used methods is the Wassermann test used in the diagnosis of syphilis. This reaction depends upon the fixation of complement by the patient's antibody after it has reacted with cardiolipin, an alcoholic extract (a phosphatide lipoid) from normal animal tissues, usually ox heart. Why antibodies against this material develop in syphilis is not clear. Some workers suggest that it results from autoimmunization with host lipids made antigenic in some way by the spirochaete (*Trep. pallidum*) responsible for syphilis whilst others believe that the spirochaete contains a cell wall antigen related to the tissue antigen (p. 16). Interpretation of the results of the Wassermann test is difficult and a final assessment depends on the results of both this and other serological tests and the clinical findings. False positive reactions are sometimes found in leprosy, malaria, sleeping sickness, tuberculosis and other febrile diseases. When there is doubt a more specific test may have to be employed – the treponemal immobilization test, in which motile treponemata can be seen to be immobilized when examined microscopically after exposure to patient's serum.

Complement fixation tests are used widely in the diagnosis of virus diseases. The source of the antigen is usually the infected tissues of animals, or eggs, or infected tissue cultures. The virus is usually extracted from the tissues or cells by differential centri-fugation or sometimes by purifying the virus by adsorbing it on to red cells and then eluting it later.

Haemagglutination-inhibition tests

Another useful procedure for the diagnosis of some types of virus disease is the 'haemagglutination-inhibition test'. This depends on the fact that certain viruses, e.g. those of influenza, mumps and parainfluenza will agglutinate chicken, human and guinea-pig red cells (Fig. 29). Other viruses, e.g. the adenoviruses, agglutinate rat or monkey red cells; the reoviruses and many enteroviruses agglutinate human red cells. The test is performed by mixing the virus with the appropriate red cells in the presence of patient's serum. If antibodies to the virus are present the virus will be unable to bring about haemagglutination. These tests are very valuable because of their extreme specificity and their ability to distinguish antibodies to various substrains and variants of viruses, e.g. the influenza virus. The complement fixation test on the other hand is less valuable for detecting these fine differences.

FURTHER READING

Campbell, D. H., Garvey Justine, S., Cremer, Natilie E. & Sussdorf, D. (1963). *Methods in Immunology*. New York: Benjamin.

Cruickshank, R. (1965). *Medical Microbiology*. Edinburgh: Livingstone.

Humphrey, J. H. & White, R. G. (1969). *Immunology for Students of Medicine*, p. 348. Oxford: Blackwell.

Nairn, R. C. (1969). *Fluorescent Protein Tracing*, 3rd ed. Edinburgh: Livingstone.

Nowotny, A. (1969). *Basic Exercises in Immunochemistry*. Berlin: Springer.

Weir, D. M. (1967). *Handbook of Experimental Immunology*. Oxford: Blackwell.

Wilkinson, A. E. (1970). The positive Wassermann reaction; investigation and interpretation. *Br. J. hosp. Med.* **4,** 47.

Williams, C. A. & Chase, M. W. (1968). *Methods in Immunology and Immunochemistry*. New York: Academic Press.

Wright, R. W. (1970). The Australia (hepatitis) antigen. *Br. J. hosp. Med.* **4,** 75.

INDEX

ABO groups, and blood transfusion, 119
Adaptive immunity, 3
Agammaglobulinaemia, 65
  Swiss type, 66
Age, influence on innate immunity, 5
Agglutination, antigen/antibody, 133, 138
  applications, 139
  by immunoglobulins, 47
  tests, diagnostic applications, 147
Agranulocytosis, 113
Allergy, definition, 69
Alum, 28
Alveolitis, allergic, immunity, 100
Amino acids, determinants of antigenic specificity, 19–20
Anaemia, acquired haemolytic, 106, 107
  autoimmune haemolytic, 113
Anaphylaxis, 70
  and allergic alveolitis, 100
  antibodies involved, 72
  pharmacological mediators, 71
  prevention, immunology, 73
    blocking antibody, 73
  shock, 71
  systemic and local forms, 72
Anaphylotoxins, 13, 71
Antibody/ies and anaphylactic reactions, 72
  role of IgE, 72
  antigen interaction, 131–149
  see also Antigen/antibody interaction
  anti-Rh, 121
  as consequence of tissue damage, 115
  blocking, 73

circulating, role in graft rejection, 85
mediated immunity in bacterial infections, 91
and non-antibody lymphocyte factors, locally produced, role in graft rejection, 86
production, cells concerned, 49
  cellular processes, 52
  and gut-associated lymphoid tissue, 58
  humoral, involvement of lymphoid tissue, 37
  theories, directive, 53
    implications and variations, 55
  selective, 54
reaginic, 72, 73
response, humoral, 25
Antigen/antibody interaction, 131–149
  agglutination, 138
  cytotoxic test, 147
  diagnostic applications, 147
  immunoelectrophoresis, 137
  optimal proportions, 133
  primary union, 132
  secondary effects, interpretation and applications, 132
Antigen-antibody reactions, 69
  using fluorescent labels, 144
Antigen(s), 15–22
  ABO, 118
  altered, 109
  alum-precipitated, 28
  anaphylactic reaction, 70
  aromatic amino acids, 17
  blood group substances, 18
  of blood leucocytes and platelets, 123
  cell-associated, cytolytic reactions, 75

151